Analysis of Data from Randomized Controlled Trials

Jos W. R. Twisk

Analysis of Data from Randomized Controlled Trials

A Practical Guide

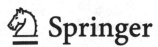

Jos W. R. Twisk
Amsterdam UMC
Amsterdam, The Netherlands

ISBN 978-3-030-81867-8   ISBN 978-3-030-81865-4   (eBook)
https://doi.org/10.1007/978-3-030-81865-4

This Springer imprint is published by the registered company Springer Nature Switzerland AG.
The registered company address is: Gewerbestrasse 11, 6330 Cham, Switzerland

To my family and friends

Contents

Chapter 1
Introduction

1.1 Introduction

Randomized controlled trials (RCTs) are considered to be the gold standard for evaluating the effect of an intervention (Rothman & Greenland, 1998). In an RCT, the population under study is randomly divided into an intervention group and a control group. Subjects in the intervention group are allocated to the intervention (e.g., a new treatment, medication, vaccination program, etc.), while subjects in the control group are allocated to the control condition (e.g., placebo, usual care, etc.). In general, an RCT starts with a baseline measurement before the intervention is started. Then, during or after the intervention period, one or more follow-up measurement is performed. Regarding the analysis of RCT data, a distinction must be made between studies with only one follow-up measurement and studies with more than one follow-up measurement. When there is only one follow-up measurement, relatively simple statistical methods can be used to estimate the effect of the intervention, while when more than one follow-up measurement is considered, in general, more advanced statistical methods are necessary.

In the past decade, an RCT with only one follow-up measurement has become rare. At least one short-term follow-up measurement and one long-term follow-up measurement "must" be performed. More than two follow-up measurements are usually performed in order to investigate the development of the outcome variable over time and to compare the developments of the outcome variable among the intervention and control groups. Sometimes these more complicated experimental designs are analyzed with simple cross-sectional methods, mostly by analyzing the outcome at each follow-up measurement separately or sometimes even by ignoring the information gathered from the in-between measurements, i.e., only using the last measurement as outcome variable to estimate the effect of the intervention. Besides this, summary statistics are sometimes used. The general idea behind a summary statistic is to capture the longitudinal development of an outcome variable over time into one value: the summary statistic. With a relative simple cross-sectional analysis,

J. W. R. Twisk, *Analysis of Data from Randomized Controlled Trials*,
https://doi.org/10.1007/978-3-030-81865-4_1

these summary statistics can be compared between the intervention and control groups in order to estimate the effect of the intervention (Twisk, 2013). However, nowadays mostly more advanced statistical methods are used to analyze RCT data with more than one follow-up measurement. In this book, the different possibilities to analyze RCT data will be discussed by using different example datasets. Different chapters will focus on different designs, such as RCTs with one follow-up measurement (Chap. 2), RCTs with more than one follow-up measurement (Chap. 3), cluster RCTs (Chap. 4), cross-over trials (Chap. 5), stepped wedge trials (Chap. 6), and N-of-1 trials (Chap. 7). In the first part of this book, all methods will be illustrated with continuous outcome variables. In Chap. 8, the differences in statistical analyses between RCTs with a continuous and a dichotomous outcome variable will be discussed. In the last part of the book, several other aspects regarding the analysis of RCT data will be discussed. These aspects include the problem what to do when only a baseline measurement is available (Chap. 9), sample size calculations (Chap. 10), and the myths of testing for baseline differences and the analysis of within group changes within an RCT (Chap. 11).

1.2   Intention-to-Treat Analysis

The standard method to estimate treatment effects in an RCT is an intention-to-treat analysis. In an intention-to-treat analysis, all subjects randomized into the intervention group should be analyzed as having received the intervention, regardless of whether they received the complete intervention, only part of the intervention, or nothing at all.

In a per protocol analysis, a comparison is made between subjects that actually followed the protocol. A per protocol analysis is often performed when the intention-to-treat analysis showed an intervention effect which is less strong than expected. When a stronger intervention effect is observed in the per protocol analysis compared to the intention-to-treat analysis it indicates that the intervention basically works, but there are probably some issues with the implementation of the intervention.

An as treated analysis is slightly different from a per protocol analysis. For instance, subjects from the intervention group who actually received the control condition are analyzed in the control group in an as treated analysis, while they are removed from the analysis in the per protocol analysis.

In general, the choice for an intention-to-treat analysis, a per protocol analysis or an as treated analysis does not influence the choice for the statistical methods that can be used to estimate the intervention effect. It only defines the population to be analyzed, and, therefore, a detailed discussion about these different populations goes beyond the scope of this book.

1.3   General Purpose and Prior Knowledge

This book will follow a practical nonmathematical approach, which will make it easier to read and more understandable for nonmathematical readers. Therefore, in each chapter, the statistical analyses will be explained by using relatively simple examples, accompanied by computer output.

The book provides a practical guide about the different ways to estimate the effect of an intervention in an RCT. It is assumed that the researchers who are going to use the book have performed a certain kind of RCT (or are planning to perform one) and that they know what kind of data they have (or going to have). This book offers an answer to the question how to estimate the intervention effect in an appropriate way, and this question will be answered for different RCT designs. In this book an attempt has been made to keep the description of the statistical analyses as simple as possible. However, it will be assumed that the reader has some prior knowledge about standard statistical regression techniques, such as linear regression analysis and logistic regression analysis.

1.4   Examples and Software

In all examples presented in this book, the statistical program STATA (version 15) was used for performing the analyses (StataCorp, 2017). All example datasets used in this book are available on request. The same holds for the STATA codes used for performing the statistical analyses on the example datasets. All can be requested by jwr.twisk@amsterdamumc.nl. It should be noted that all analyses can also be performed with other software programs such as R, SPSS, and SAS. In general, the syntax to be used is not that difficult.

1.5   Equations

In the different chapters, several equations are used to explain the methods used to analyze the data. Because this book is written for the nonmathematical researcher, these equations are printed in a relative simple way. Again, this is done to make the book easily accessible for readers without a mathematical or statistical background.

Chapter 2
Analysis of RCT Data with One Follow-Up Measurement

2.1 Statistical Methods

When the effect of an intervention is estimated in an RCT with a continuous outcome variable and only one follow-up measurement, mostly the change between the baseline measurement and the follow-up measurement in the continuous outcome variable is compared between the intervention group and the control group. The effect of the intervention can then be estimated with a linear regression analysis (Eq. 2.1) or even by an independent t-test. An independent t-test is basically the same as a linear regression analysis with a dichotomous independent variable, i.e., the intervention variable:

$$\Delta Y_t = Y_{t1} - Y_{t0} \tag{2.1a}$$

$$\Delta Y_t = \beta_0 + \beta_1 X \tag{2.1b}$$

where Y_{t0} = outcome measured at baseline, Y_{t1} = outcome measured at follow-up, X = intervention variable, and β_1 = effect estimate.

Comparing the change between the baseline measurement and the follow-up measurement is a very popular method to analyze RCT data with one follow-up measurement, because it greatly reduces the complexity of the statistical analysis. However, the analysis of the change score is more problematic than is usually realized.

One of the typical problems related to the use of the change score is the phenomenon of regression to the mean. If the outcome variable at baseline is a sample of random numbers and the outcome variable at the follow-up measurement is also a sample of random numbers, then the subjects in the upper part of the distribution at baseline are less likely to be in the upper part of the distribution at the follow-up measurement, compared to the other subjects. In the same way, the subjects in the lower part of the distribution at baseline are less likely to be in the

© The Author(s), under exclusive license to Springer Nature Switzerland AG 2021
J. W. R. Twisk, *Analysis of Data from Randomized Controlled Trials*,
https://doi.org/10.1007/978-3-030-81865-4_2

Fig. 2.1 Regression to the
mean in one population

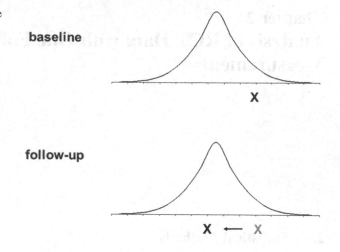

lower part of the distribution at the follow-up measurement compared to the other subjects (see Fig. 2.1).

When the change over time in a whole population is analyzed, regression to the mean is not really a big problem, because in one population there will be subjects with a random increase, and there will be subjects with a random decrease. So, on average, there will be no change. However, in an RCT, when two groups are compared to each other, regression to the mean can be a big problem, which occurs when the average baseline values of the outcome variable differs between the two groups.

The general idea of an RCT is that the two groups are randomly allocated to either the intervention group or the control group. Because of this random allocation, it is assumed that at baseline the average values of the two groups are the same. However, that is theoretically only the case when the size of the (source) population is infinite. In a real-life RCT, however, the two groups are of limited size, and therefore it is highly possible that the average baseline values of the outcome variable differ between the two groups. When the two groups are derived from one (source) population, this difference is totally caused by chance. Suppose that the aim of a particular intervention is to decrease the outcome variable, and suppose further that the intervention group has a higher average baseline value compared to the control group; when the intervention has no effect at all, due to regression to the mean, the average value of the intervention group will go down, while the average value of the control group will go up. A comparison between the intervention and the control group regarding the change over time (Eq. 2.1) will then reveal a favorable intervention effect. This is not a "real" effect but an effect caused by regression to the mean (see Fig. 2.2).

Some researchers believe that using the relative change (Eq. 2.2) adjusts for regression to the mean. However, that is not the case. In Fig. 2.3, this is nicely illustrated:

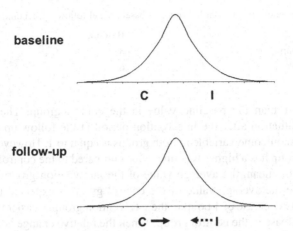

Fig. 2.2 Influence of regression to the mean on the estimation of an intervention effect in an RCT (I = intervention group; C = control group)

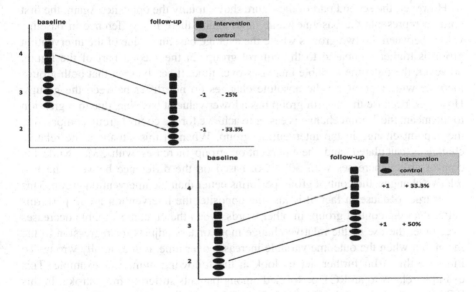

Fig. 2.3 The use of a relative change (Eq. 2.2) does not adjusts for regression to the mean

$$\Delta Y_{rel} = \frac{(Y_{t1} - Y_{t0})}{Y_{t0}} \times 100\% \qquad (2.2a)$$

$$\Delta Y_{rel} = \beta_0 + \beta_1 X \qquad (2.2b)$$

where Y_{t0} = outcome measured at baseline, Y_{t1} = outcome measured at follow-up, X = intervention variable, and β_1 = effect estimate.

In Fig. 2.3, two situations are illustrated. In the first situation, the first column represents the baseline value. It can be seen that the baseline value in the intervention

Table 2.1 Mean values for the Barthel Index at baseline and follow-up; a numerical example

	Baseline	Follow-up
Intervention group ($N = 40$)	8	16
Control group ($N = 40$)	6	12

group is higher than the baseline value in the control group. The next column indicates the situation after the intervention period at the follow-up measurement. The decrease in outcome variable in both groups is equal to 1. However, because the intervention group has a higher baseline value compared to the control group, due to regression to the mean, the average value of the intervention group is expected to decrease, while the average value of the control group is expected to increase. In other words, the decrease of 1 point in the intervention group is easier to achieve than the 1 point decrease in the control group. When the relative change is calculated, the intervention group decreases with 25%, while the control group decreases with 33%. So, in this situation (when there is a decrease in the outcome variable), the use of the relative change works well.

However, the second part of the figure shows totally the opposite. Again, the first column represents the baseline value, and, again, there is a difference in baseline values between the two groups where the average baseline value of the intervention group is higher compared to the control group. In the second part of the figure, however, the outcome variable increases over time. It can be seen that both groups increase with 1 point, so the absolute changes do not differ between the groups. However, because the control group has a lower value at baseline, due to regression to the mean, the 1 point change is easier to achieve for the control group compared to the 1 point change in the intervention group. When in this situation, the relative change is calculated, and the intervention group increases with 33%, while the control group increases with 50%. So, based on the difference between the two relative changes, the control group performs better than the intervention group. This is not true, because in fact, it is just the opposite; the intervention group performs better than the control group. In other words, when the outcome variable decreases over time, the use of the relative change more or less adjusts for regression to the mean, but when the outcome variable increases over time, it goes totally wrong. To illustrate this a bit further, let us look at the following numerical example. This example relates to an RCT performed among patients suffering from stroke. In this RCT the outcome was the Barthel Index, which indicates the possibility to perform regular activities of daily living, such as standing up from a chair, taking a shower, etc. Table 2.1 shows the data of this numerical example.

From Table 2.1 it is obvious that the baseline values differ between the two groups. The intervention group has a higher baseline value compared to the control group. Because there is an increase in the outcome variable over time, the increase of 8 points for the intervention group is harder to achieve than the increase of 6 points for the control group. The control group is helped by regression to the mean, while the intervention group is counteracted by regression to the mean. So, the difference between the two groups of 2 points in change over time is an underestimation of the actual effect of the intervention. When the relative change is calculated for both groups, there is an increase of 100% for both groups, which indicates that the intervention does not work at all. This example shows nicely that analyzing the relative change does not adjusts for regression to the mean. So, it can be concluded that the method of comparing relative change scores should not be used in the analysis of RCT data with one follow-up measurement.

Another method that claims to adjust for regression to the mean is known as analysis of covariance (Eq. 2.3). With this method the value of the outcome variable Y at the follow-up measurement is used as outcome in a linear regression analysis, while the baseline value of the outcome variable Y is added to the model as a covariate:

$$Y_{t1} = \beta_0 + \beta_1 X + \beta_2 Y_{t0} \tag{2.3}$$

where Y_{t1} = outcome measured at follow-up, Y_{t0} = outcome measured at baseline, X = intervention variable, β_1 = effect estimate, and β_2 = regression coefficient for the baseline value.

In this model, β_1 indicates the effect of the intervention adjusted for possible differences at baseline, i.e., adjusted for regression to the mean. In the analysis of covariance, the regression coefficient for the baseline value (β_2) is known as the autoregression coefficient. The analysis is comparable to the analysis of residual change, which was first described by Blomquist (1977). The first step in the analysis of residual change is to perform a linear regression analysis between Y_{t1} and Y_{t0}. The second step is to calculate the difference between the observed value of Y_{t1} and the predicted value of Y_{t1} (predicted by the regression model with Y_{t0}). This difference is called the residual change, which is then used as outcome variable in a linear regression analysis with the intervention variable. The regression coefficient of the intervention variable is an estimate of the effect of the intervention adjusting for regression to the mean. Although the general idea behind residual change analysis is the same as for analysis of covariance, the results of both methods are not exactly the same. From the literature it is known that analysis of residual change is not as good as analysis of covariance (Forbes & Carlin, 2005). So, the analysis of residual change will not be considered any further in the remaining part of this book.

Some researchers argue that the best way to define changes, adjusting for regression to the mean, is a combination of Eqs. (2.1) and (2.3). They suggest to use the change between the baseline measurement and the follow-up measurement as outcome in a linear regression analysis, adjusting for the baseline value of the outcome (Eq. 2.4):

$$Y_{t1} - Y_{t0} = \beta_0 + \beta_1 X + \beta_2 Y_{t0} \tag{2.4}$$

where Y_{t1} = outcome measured at follow-up, Y_{t0} = outcome measured at baseline, X = intervention variable, β_1 = effect estimate, and β_2 = regression coefficient for the baseline value.

However, analyzing the change, adjusting for the baseline value, is exactly the same as the analysis of covariance described in Eq. (2.3). The only difference between the models is that the regression coefficient for the baseline value is

Table 2.2 Data structure needed to perform an analysis of changes and an analysis of covariance

Id	Outcome 1[a]	Outcome 2[b]	Intervention	Baseline
1	Y_{t1}	$Y_{t1} - Y_{t0}$	1	Y_{t0}
2	Y_{t1}	$Y_{t1} - Y_{t0}$	1	Y_{t0}
3	Y_{t1}	$Y_{t1} - Y_{t0}$	0	Y_{t0}

[a]Outcome used for the analysis of covariance
[b]Outcome used for the analysis of changes

different, i.e., the difference between the regression coefficients for the baseline value is equal to 1. See Box 2.1 for a detailed explanation.

Boxspiepr146 2.1

Mathematical equivalence between analysis of covariance and the analysis of changes with an adjustment for the baseline value of the outcome

Analysis of covariance	Analysis of changes with adjustment for the baseline value
$Y_{t1} = \beta_0 + \beta_1 X + \beta_2 Y_{t0}$	$Y_{t1} - Y_{t0} = \beta_0 + \beta_1 X + \beta_2 Y_{t0}$
	$Y_{t1} = \beta_0 + \beta_1 X + \beta_2 Y_{t0} + Y_{t0}$
	$Y_{t1} = \beta_0 + \beta_1 X + (1 + \beta_2) Y_{t0}$

When the equation of analysis of changes is rewritten to define the outcome Y_{t1}, only the regression coefficient of Y_{t0} changes by a value of 1. The coefficient of the intervention variable remains the same. So, whether Y_{t1} or $Y_{t1} - Y_{t0}$ is being used as an outcome, the effect estimate will be exactly the same.

Table 2.2 shows the structure of the data used to estimate the parameters for the different analyses.

2.2   Example

The example dataset used in this chapter is derived from an RCT among 299 civil servants working within municipal services in the Netherlands (Proper et al., 2003; Twisk & Proper, 2004). All subjects randomized into the intervention group were offered seven consultations, each 20 min in duration. The intervention period was 9 months, and counseling was focused primarily on the enhancement of the individual's level of physical activity. Subjects in the control group received no individual counseling. Outcome variables were measured at baseline and directly after the completion of the last consultation.

In principle, the RCT had three primary outcome variables (physical activity, cardiorespiratory fitness, and prevalence of musculoskeletal disorders [e.g., upper extremity complaints]) and three secondary outcomes (body composition [i.e., the percentage of body fat and the body mass index], blood pressure, and total serum cholesterol), but to make the example not too extensive, we selected two continuous

Table 2.3 Mean and standard deviation (in parentheses) for the outcome variables used in the example, i.e., total serum cholesterol and the physical activity index

		Baseline	Follow-up
Total serum Cholesterol (mmol/l)	Intervention group (*N* = 105)	5.52 (1.03)	5.35 (0.99
	Control group (*N* = 117)	5.33 (0.91)	5.33 (0.93)
Physical activity index	Intervention group (*N* = 99)	5.80 (1.07)	5.94 (0.95)
	Control group (*N* = 118)	5.44 (1.09)	5.34 (1.05)

```
    Source |       SS           df       MS              Number of obs   =      222
-----------+------------------------------------         F(1, 220)       =     4.68
     Model |  1.80405499          1  1.80405499          Prob > F        =   0.0317
  Residual |  84.8837288        220  .385835131          R-squared       =   0.0208
-----------+------------------------------------         Adj R-squared   =   0.0164
     Total |  86.6877838        221  .392252415          Root MSE        =   .62116


-----------------------------------------------------------------------------------
   delchol |      Coef.   Std. Err.      t    P>|t|     [95% Conf. Interval]
-----------+-----------------------------------------------------------------------
   interven |  -.1805568   .0835006   -2.16   0.032    -.3451203   -.0159933
      _cons |   .0051282   .0574259    0.09   0.929    -.1080471    .1183035
-----------------------------------------------------------------------------------
```

Output 2.1 Result of the linear regression analysis comparing the changes in total serum cholesterol from baseline to follow-up between the intervention and control groups

```
    Source |       SS           df       MS              Number of obs   =      222
-----------+------------------------------------         F(2, 219)       =    17.12
     Model |  11.7218792          2  5.86093961          Prob > F        =   0.0000
  Residual |  74.9659046        219  .342310067          R-squared       =   0.1352
-----------+------------------------------------         Adj R-squared   =   0.1273
     Total |  86.6877838        221  .392252415          Root MSE        =   .58507


-----------------------------------------------------------------------------------
   delchol |      Coef.   Std. Err.      t    P>|t|     [95% Conf. Interval]
-----------+-----------------------------------------------------------------------
   interven |  -.1374189   .0790573   -1.74   0.084    -.2932293    .0183915
    t0chol |  -.2190814   .0407012   -5.38   0.000    -.2992975   -.1388652
      _cons |   1.172008   .2234304    5.25   0.000     .7316589    1.612357
-----------------------------------------------------------------------------------
```

Output 2.2 Result of the linear regression analysis comparing the changes in total serum cholesterol from baseline to follow-up between the intervention and control groups adjusted for the baseline value

outcome variables (physical activity and total serum cholesterol), which were selected because of differences between the groups at baseline (see Table 2.3). Physical activity was assessed by the Baecke questionnaire. With this questionnaire, physical activities during sport and during leisure time were measured. Both were combined into one physical activity index.

From Table 2.3 it can be seen that for both the physical activity index and total serum cholesterol, the baseline value for the intervention group is higher than for the control group.

To analyze the effect of the intervention, three methods were used which were all described in Sect. 2.1: (1) the comparison of changes (Eq. 2.1); (2) the comparison of

```
  Source |       SS            df       MS           Number of obs   =        222
---------+------------------------------------       F(2, 219)       =     184.09
   Model |  126.028315          2   63.0141576       Prob > F        =     0.0000
Residual |  74.9659046        219   .342310067       R-squared       =     0.6270
---------+------------------------------------       Adj R-squared   =     0.6236
   Total |   200.99422        221   .909476108       Root MSE        =     .58507


   t1chol |     Coef.   Std. Err.      t    P>|t|     [95% Conf. Interval]
---------+------------------------------------------------------------------
 interven |  -.1374189   .0790573    -1.74   0.084    -.2932293     .0183915
   t0chol |   .7809186   .0407012    19.19   0.000     .7007025     .8611348
    _cons |   1.172008   .2234304     5.25   0.000     .7316589     1.612357
```

Output 2.3 Result of the analysis of covariance for total serum cholesterol

changes, adjusted for the baseline value (Eq. 2.4); and (3) the analysis of covariance (Eq. 2.3). Outputs 2.1–2.3 show the results for total serum cholesterol.

In all three analyses reported in Outputs 2.1–2.3, the regression coefficient for the intervention variable indicates the effect of the intervention. It can be seen that the effect of the intervention is stronger when the changes from baseline to follow-up are analyzed without adjustment for the baseline value (-0.18 versus -0.14). The stronger effect estimate, however, is an overestimation of the "real" intervention effect. This overestimation is caused by the differences between the groups at baseline. Because the intervention group starts at a higher level, and the intervention is intending to decrease total serum cholesterol values, regression to the mean tends the intervention group to decrease. Analysis of covariance adjusts for the differences at baseline, and therefore this analysis showed a less strong intervention effect. As has been explained in Box 2.1, the analysis of covariance and the analysis of changes adjusted for the baseline value provide the same intervention effect. The only difference between the two methods is that the autoregression coefficient (i.e., the regression coefficient for the baseline value) differs by the value of 1. Based on these results, it can be concluded that the "real" intervention effect equals -0.14. This indicates that at the follow-up measurement, total serum cholesterol is 0.14 mmol/liter lower for the intervention group compared to the control group. Besides this, it can also be seen that the 95% confidence interval around the difference ranges between -0.29 and 0.02, with a corresponding p-value of 0.084.

Although for both total serum cholesterol and the physical activity index the intervention group has higher values at baseline, for the physical activity index, the results of the three analyses show a different picture than for total serum cholesterol (see Outputs 2.4–2.6).

From Outputs 2.4–2.6 it can be seen that the analysis of changes now underestimates the effect of the intervention. Again this is due to the differences at baseline between the intervention and the control group. However, in contrast to total serum cholesterol, the intervention intended to increase physical activity instead of to decrease. When an increase is expected, for the group with the highest average value at baseline (i.e., the intervention group), the increase is harder to achieve than the increase for the group with the lower average value at baseline (i.e., the control group). Therefore, the adjustment for the baseline value leads to a higher intervention effect (0.35 versus 0.24). So, the "real" intervention effect indicates that at the

```
      Source |       SS           df       MS            Number of obs   =      217
-------------+--------------------------------            F(1, 215)       =     6.27
       Model |   3.2266743         1    3.2266743         Prob > F        =   0.0130
    Residual |  110.703625       215   .514900582         R-squared       =   0.0283
-------------+--------------------------------            Adj R-squared   =   0.0238
       Total |   113.9303        216   .52745509          Root MSE        =   .71757


      delact |    Coef.    Std. Err.      t     P>|t|     [95% Conf. Interval]
-------------+----------------------------------------------------------------
     interven |  .2448211   .0977987     2.50   0.013     .0520541    .4375881
        _cons | -.1059322   .0660573    -1.60   0.110    -.236135     .0242706
```

Output 2.4 Result of the linear regression analysis comparing the changes in the physical activity index from baseline to follow-up between the intervention and control groups

```
      Source |       SS           df       MS            Number of obs   =      217
-------------+--------------------------------            F(2, 214)       =    28.54
       Model |  23.9875439         2   11.993772          Prob > F        =   0.0000
    Residual |  89.9427556       214   .420293251         R-squared       =   0.2105
-------------+--------------------------------            Adj R-squared   =   0.2032
       Total |   113.9303        216   .52745509          Root MSE        =    .6483


      delact |    Coef.    Std. Err.      t     P>|t|     [95% Conf. Interval]
-------------+----------------------------------------------------------------
     interven |  .3473814   .0895552     3.88   0.000     .1708581    .5239047
       t0act | -.2867148   .0407947    -7.03   0.000    -.3671256   -.2063039
        _cons |  1.454598   .229918      6.33   0.000     1.001404    1.907792
```

Output 2.5 Result of the linear regression analysis comparing the changes in the physical activity index from baseline to follow-up between the intervention and control groups adjusted for the baseline value

```
      Source |       SS           df       MS            Number of obs   =      217
-------------+--------------------------------            F(2, 214)       =   176.11
       Model |  148.034779         2   74.0173895         Prob > F        =   0.0000
    Residual |  89.9427556       214   .420293251         R-squared       =   0.6221
-------------+--------------------------------            Adj R-squared   =   0.6185
       Total |  237.977535       216   1.10174785         Root MSE        =    .6483


       t1act |    Coef.    Std. Err.      t     P>|t|     [95% Conf. Interval]
-------------+----------------------------------------------------------------
     interven |  .3473814   .0895552     3.88   0.000     .1708581    .5239047
       t0act |  .7132852   .0407947    17.48   0.000     .6328744    .7936961
        _cons |  1.454598   .229918      6.33   0.000     1.001404    1.907792
```

Output 2.6 Result of the analysis of covariance for the physical activity index

follow-up measurement, the physical activity index is 0.35 units higher in the intervention group compared to the control group. The 95% confidence interval around this difference ranges between 0.17 and 0.52, with a corresponding p-value <0.001.

Chapter 3
Analysis of RCT Data with More Than One Follow-Up Measurement

3.1 Introduction

In Chap. 2, the analysis of data from an RCT with only one follow-up measurement was discussed. However, as has been mentioned before, in the past decade, an RCT with only one follow-up measurement has become very rare. Mostly more than one follow-up measurement is performed. In some RCTs two follow-up measurements are performed in order to estimate the short-term and long-term effects of the intervention, but sometimes even more follow-up measurements are performed in order to estimate the difference in the development over time in a particular outcome between the intervention and control groups.

Basically, for the analysis of data from an RCT with more than one follow-up measurement, the same problems arise than for the analysis of data from an RCT with only one follow-up measurement, i.e., an adjustment must be made for the baseline value in order to adjust for regression to the mean. Until the start of a new millennium, the analyses of data from an RCT with more than one follow-up measurement were split into separate parts, i.e., the effect of the intervention was estimated for all follow-up measurements separately. Although it is interesting to estimate the intervention effects at the different follow-up measurements, performing separate analyses for the different follow-up measurements ignores the fact that the measurements were performed on the same subjects, i.e., it ignores the fact that the repeated measurements on the same subject are dependent of each other. Because of that, nowadays, it is necessary to take this dependency of the observations into account and estimate the effects of the intervention at different follow-up measurements in one statistical model. The most classical way to do this is to use a generalized linear model (GLM) for repeated measures, but that method has some serious flaws. Therefore, regression-based methods such as mixed models or generalized estimating equations (GEE analysis) are mostly used to estimate the effect of an intervention from an RCT with more than one follow-up measurement. In the remaining part of this chapter, several methods will be discussed that can be used

J. W. R. Twisk, *Analysis of Data from Randomized Controlled Trials*,
https://doi.org/10.1007/978-3-030-81865-4_3

(or are used) in the analysis of RCT data with more than one follow-up measurement. Not all of the methods are equally appropriate for the analysis of RCT data with more than one follow-up measurement, but it is important to discuss the pros and cons of the different methods to finally give a solid recommendation which method (s) should be used.

3.2 Example

To illustrate the different possible ways to analysis RCT data with more than one follow-up measurement, a hypothetical example will be used. In this example dataset, a new intervention is compared to a control condition regarding the outcome variable complaints. Complaints are measured as a continuous outcome variable, and beside a baseline measurement, three follow-up measurements were performed. Table 3.1 shows descriptive information for both the intervention and control groups at all four measurements.

3.3 GLM for Repeated Measures

The basic idea behind GLM for repeated measures (which is also known as (multivariate) analysis of variance ((M)ANOVA) for repeated measures) is the same as for the well-known paired t-test. Within a GLM for repeated measures, the statistical testing is carried out for the $T - 1$ absolute differences between subsequent measurements. In fact, GLM for repeated measures is a multivariate analysis of these $T - 1$ absolute differences. Multivariate refers to the fact that $T - 1$ differences are used simultaneously as outcome variable. Besides the multivariate approach, the same research question can also be answered with a univariate approach. This univariate procedure is comparable to the procedures carried out in an analysis of variance (ANOVA) and is based on the sum of squares, i.e., squared differences between observed values and average values. From a GLM for repeated measures with one dichotomous independent variable (i.e., the intervention variable), basically three effects can be derived: an overall time effect (i.e., is there a change over time, independent of the different groups), an overall group effect (i.e., is there a difference between the groups on average over time) and, most important, a group-time interaction effect (i.e., is there a difference between the groups in development

	Intervention group	Control group
Baseline	3.25 (0.40)	3.47 (0.43)
1st follow-up	3.03 (0.45)	3.25 (0.48)
2nd follow-up	2.89 (0.51)	3.18 (0.57)
3rd follow-up	2.83 (0.47)	3.12 (0.55)

Table 3.1 Descriptive information (mean and standard deviation) of the outcome variable complaints

Table 3.2 Data structure needed to perform a GLM for repeated measures

id	Outcome	Time	Intervention	Baseline[a]
1	Y_{t0}	0	1	Y_{t0}
1	Y_{t1}	1	1	Y_{t0}
1	Y_{t2}	2	1	Y_{t0}
1	Y_{t3}	3	1	Y_{t0}

Note: in some software packages (such as SPSS), a broad data structure is needed to perform a GLM for repeated measures
[a]Because the baseline value is also used as outcome, a copy value is needed

```
              Number of obs =        572    R-squared     =  0.7006
              Root MSE      =  .336569    Adj R-squared =  0.5830

        Source | Partial SS         df          MS          F     Prob>F
---------------+------------------------------------------------------------
         Model | 108.67927         161      .6750265       5.96   0.0000
               |
    intervent~n | 8.486801           1      8.486801      15.11   0.0002
patnr|intervent~n | 86.485301       154      .56159286
---------------+------------------------------------------------------------
          time | 12.84741           3      4.28247       37.80   0.0000
 intervent~n#time | .20660739        3      .06886913      0.61   0.6101
               |
      Residual | 46.444287         410      .11327875
---------------+------------------------------------------------------------
         Total | 155.12355         571      .27166997
```

Output 3.1 Results of a GLM for repeated measures performed on the example dataset

over time). See for details, regarding GLM for repeated measures, Twisk et al. (2013). Table 3.2 shows the structure of the data used to estimate the parameters of a GLM for repeated measures.

Output 3.1 shows the results of a GLM for repeated measures performed on the example dataset, while Fig. 3.1 shows the so-called estimated marginal means resulting from the GLM for repeated measures.

Output 3.1 contains two tables with results. The first table of the results shows the p-value for the overall intervention effect ($p = 0.0002$). This highly significant p-value indicates the difference between the intervention group and the control group on average over time. In the second table of the results, the p-values are given for the overall time effect ($p < 0.001$) and for the interaction between intervention and time ($p = 0.6101$). The overall time effect indicates the development over time for the whole population, while the intervention-time interaction effect indicates the difference in development over time between the intervention and control groups. From Fig. 3.1 and Table 3.1, however, it can be seen that the baseline values of both groups are different. In Chap. 2 it was already discussed that the difference in baseline values between the groups leads to regression to the mean and that, therefore, an adjustment must be made for these baseline differences. Within the framework of a GLM for repeated measures, also an adjustment can be made for the baseline value. This approach is also known as a multivariate analysis of covariance (MANCOVA) for repeated measures. Output 3.2 and Fig. 3.2 show the results of a

Fig. 3.1 Estimated
marginal means derived
from a GLM for repeated
measures performed on the
example dataset (continuous
line = control; dotted line =
intervention)

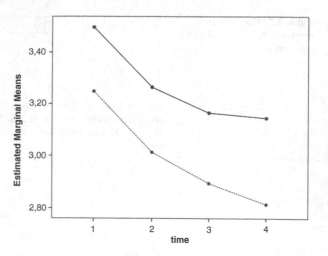

```
             Number of obs =        572    R-squared     =  0.7273
             Root MSE      =   .322412    Adj R-squared =  0.6174

        Source | Partial SS        df          MS           F     Prob>F
----------------+----------------------------------------------------------
         Model |  112.81612        164    .68790318        6.62   0.0000
               |
   intervent~n |  1.4798342          1   1.4798342         5.11   0.0252
      baseline |  .40749289          1    .40749289        1.41   0.2374
patnr|intervent~n |  44.321113      153    .28968048
----------------+----------------------------------------------------------
          time |  2.6901628          3    .89672092        8.63   0.0000
      baseline |  .40749289          1    .40749289        3.92   0.0484
intervent~n#time |  .65729745        3    .21909915        2.11   0.0987
 time#baseline |  4.1368547          3   1.3789516        13.27   0.0000
               |
      Residual |  42.307432        407    .10394946
----------------+----------------------------------------------------------
         Total |  155.12355        571    .27166997
```

Output 3.2 Results of a GLM for repeated measures adjusted for the baseline differences performed on the example dataset

GLM for repeated measures adjusting for the baseline value performed on the example dataset.

From Output 3.2 it can be seen that the p-value for the interaction between intervention and time decreases to 0.0987. The latter is a better indication of the significance level of the intervention effect, because from Fig. 3.2 it can be seen that the decrease in complaints over time is a bit in favor of the intervention group. It also makes sense in light of the adjustment for regression to the mean. Because the intervention group has a lower baseline value, the decrease in complaints is harder to achieve. An adjustment for the baseline value provided, therefore, a lower p-value for the interaction between intervention and time.

Although GLM for repeated measures is often used, it has a few major drawbacks. First of all, it can only be applied to complete cases; all subjects with one or

Fig. 3.2 Estimated marginal means derived from a GLM for repeated measures adjusted for the baseline differences performed on the example dataset (continuous line = control; dotted line = intervention)

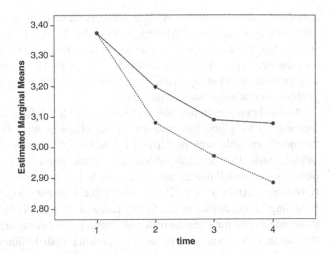

more missing observation are not part of the analyses. Secondly, GLM for repeated measures is mainly based on statistical testing. The parameters obtained from a GLM for repeated measures are p-values. This is a major drawback, because there is much more interest in effect estimates and confidence intervals around the effect estimates. Within a GLM for repeated measures, it is hard to get a proper effect estimate. Because of this, nowadays, GLM for repeated measures is not much used for the analysis of RCT data with more than one follow-up measurement.

3.4 Regression-Based Methods

The two mostly used regression-based methods to analyze RCT data with more than one follow-up measurement are mixed model analysis and GEE analysis (Twisk, 2013). The two most important advantages of the regression-based methods are that all available data is included in the analysis and that they provide effect estimates and confidence intervals around the effect estimates.

It has been mentioned before that when more than one follow-up measurement is analyzed in one statistical model, an adjustment must be made for the dependency of the repeated observations within the subject. In fact, when there is more than one follow-up measurement, there is longitudinal data. Both mixed models and GEE analysis can be used to analyze longitudinal data, and the difference between the two methods is that they take into account this dependency in a different way.

The basic idea behind the adjustment for the dependency of the observations within the subject is that in the regression model an adjustment has to be made for the variable "subject." The variable "subject" is mostly the id number, and although it looks like a discrete variable, in regression modeling, it should be treated as a categorical variable, and a categorical variable must be represented by dummy variables. Suppose there are 200 subjects in a particular RCT; this means that 199 dummy variables are needed to adjust for "subject." Because this is practically impossible, the adjustment for "subject" has to be performed in a more efficient way, and the two regression-based methods that are mostly used to analyze longitudinal data (mixed model analysis and GEE analysis) differ from each other in the way they perform that adjustment (Twisk, 2013).

As has been mentioned before, the general idea behind all longitudinal statistical methods is to adjust for "subject" in an efficient way. If the adjustment for the "subject" variable was performed by adding dummy variables to the regression model, basically for each subject a separate intercept is estimated. The starting point of a mixed model analysis, which is also known as multilevel analysis (Goldstein, 2003; Twisk, 2006), hierarchical linear modeling, or random effects modeling (Fitzmaurice et al., 2004; Laird & Ware, 1982), is the estimation of all these intercepts, but then the different intercepts are summarized into one coefficient: the variance. This variance is based on a normal distribution that is drawn over all the intercepts. So, a mixed model analysis consists of three steps: (1) estimating the different intercepts for all subjects, (2) drawing a normal distribution over all these intercepts, and (3) estimating the variance of that normal distribution. That variance is known as the random intercept variance, and the random intercept variance is added to the regression model.

It is also possible that not only the intercept is different for each subject but that also the development over time is different for each subject; in other words, there is an interaction between "subject" and time. In this situation the variance of the regression coefficients for time can be estimated, i.e., a random slope for time. In fact, this kind of individual interactions (i.e., random slopes) can be added to the regression model for all independent variables that are time-dependent. In a regular RCT, however, assuming a random slope for the intervention is not possible, because the intervention variable is time-independent (Twisk, 2006). When a certain subject is assigned to either the intervention or control group, that subject stays in that group along the intervention period. An exception is the cross-over trial, in which the subject is its own control and the intervention variable is, therefore, time-dependent. In this situation the intervention effect can be different for each subject, and therefore a random slope for the intervention variable can be added to the model (see Chap. 5).

Within GEE analysis, the adjustment for the dependency of observations is done in a slightly different way, i.e., by assuming (a priori) a certain working correlation structure for the repeated measurements of the outcome variable (Liang & Zeger, 1986; Zeger & Liang, 1986). Depending on the software package used to estimate the regression coefficients, different correlation structures are available. They basically vary from an exchangeable (or compound symmetry) correlation structure, i.e., the correlations between subsequent measurements are assumed to be the same, irrespective of the length of the interval between the repeated measurements, to an unstructured correlation structure. In this structure no particular structure is assumed, which means that all possible correlations between the follow-up measurements are estimated.

In the literature it is assumed that GEE analysis is robust against a wrong choice for a correlation structure, i.e., it does not matter which correlation structure is chosen; the results of the longitudinal analysis will be more or less the same (Liang & Zeger, 1986; Twisk, 2004). However, when the results of analyses with different working correlation structures are compared to each other, the magnitude of the regression coefficients can be different (Twisk, 2013). It is therefore important to realize which correlation structure should be chosen for the analysis. Although the unstructured working correlation structure is theoretically always the best, the simplicity of the correlation structure also has to be taken into account. The number of parameters (in this case correlation coefficients) which needs to be estimated differs for the various working correlation structures. The best option is therefore to choose the simplest structure which fits the data well. The first step in choosing a certain correlation structure can be to investigate the observed within person correlation coefficients for the outcome variable. It should be kept in mind that when analyzing covariates, the correlation structure can change (i.e., the choice of the correlation structure should better be based conditionally on the covariates). For a detailed explanation of the principles behind mixed model analysis and GEE analysis, one is referred to Twisk et al. (2013).

Within the framework of the regression-based methods, several models are available to evaluate the effect of an intervention in an RCT with more than one follow-up measurement (Twisk et al., 2018). In the next part of this chapter, the different models will be discussed.

3.4.1 Longitudinal Analysis of Covariance

Longitudinal analysis of covariance is an extension of the analysis of covariance described in Chap. 2, i.e., the outcome variable measured at the different follow-up measurements is adjusted for the baseline value of the outcome (Eq. 3.1):

$$Y_t = \beta_0 + \beta_1 X + \beta_2 Y_{t0} \tag{3.1}$$

where Y_t = outcome measured at the follow-up measurements, X = intervention variable, β_1 = overall intervention effect, and Y_{t0} = outcome measured at baseline.

Table 3.3 shows the structure of the data used to estimate the parameters for a longitudinal analysis of covariance.

Output 3.3 shows the results of the longitudinal analysis of covariance (Eq. 3.1) performed with linear mixed model analysis to estimate the overall intervention effect over time in the example dataset which was introduced in Sect. 3.2.

Output 3.3 basically contains three parts. The first part shows some general information regarding the analysis which is performed. It can be seen that a mixed effects maximum likelihood (ML) regression analysis is performed and that the group variable is the id number. This means that the mixed model analysis takes into account the dependency of the observations within the subject. It can also be seen

Table 3.3 Data structure needed to perform a longitudinal analysis of covariance

Id	Outcome	Time	Intervention	Baseline
1	Y_{t1}	0	1	Y_{t0}
1	Y_{t2}	1	1	Y_{t0}
1	Y_{t3}	2	1	Y_{t0}

```
Mixed-effects ML regression                     Number of obs    =      416
Group variable: id                              Number of groups =      150

                                                Obs per group:
                                                             min =        1
                                                             avg =      2.8
                                                             max =        3

                                                Wald chi2(2)     =    58.85
Log likelihood = -223.41988                     Prob > chi2      =   0.0000

-----------------------------------------------------------------------------
 complaints |      Coef.   Std. Err.      z    P>|z|     [95% Conf. Interval]
------------+----------------------------------------------------------------
intervention|   -.1419588   .0654837    -2.17   0.030    -.2703044   -.0136132
   baseline |    .5243691   .0782574     6.70   0.000     .3709873    .6777509
      _cons |    1.356396   .2742621     4.95   0.000     .818852     1.89394
-----------------------------------------------------------------------------


-----------------------------------------------------------------------------
  Random-effects Parameters  |   Estimate   Std. Err.     [95% Conf. Interval]
-----------------------------+-----------------------------------------------
id: Identity                 |
                 var(_cons)  |   .1129856   .0182538      .0823197    .1550753
-----------------------------+-----------------------------------------------
               var(Residual) |    .104595   .0091373      .0881356    .1241282
-----------------------------------------------------------------------------
LR test vs. linear model: chibar2(01) = 92.75        Prob >= chibar2 = 0.0000
```

Output 3.3 Results of the longitudinal mixed model analysis of covariance

that there are 416 observations performed among 150 subjects and that the average number of follow-up measurements is 2.8. These numbers indicate that not all patients were measured at all follow-up measurements. It should be noted that the regression-based methods and especially mixed model analysis are highly suitable to deal with missing data (Twisk et al., 2013). Furthermore, this part of the output shows some additional model fit information, such as the log likelihood. The log likelihood is used in the likelihood ratio test, which can be used to compare models with each other.

The second part of the output contains the fixed part of the mixed model. In this part of the output, the regression coefficients are given. Besides that, also the standard errors, z-values, p-values, and 95% confidence intervals around the regression coefficients are provided. The coefficient for intervention (-0.1419588) indicates that on average over time, the intervention group has a 0.14 lower score on complaints compared to the control group. The standard error of this coefficient equals 0.0654837, and the z-value (-2.17) is derived by dividing the regression coefficient by its standard error. Based on the z-value, the p-value (0.030) is obtained, and the 95% confidence interval around the regression coefficient (-0.2703044 to -0.0136132) is calculated by the regression coefficient $\pm$ 1.96

```
GEE population-averaged model                    Number of obs    =        416
Group variable:                      id          Number of groups =        150
Link:                          identity          Obs per group:
Family:                        Gaussian                          min =          1
Correlation:               exchangeable                          avg =        2.8
                                                                 max =          3
                                                 Wald chi2(2)     =      45.40
Scale parameter:               .2142789          Prob > chi2      =     0.0000

                                  (Std. Err. adjusted for clustering on id)
------------------------------------------------------------------------------
             |               Robust
complaints   |     Coef.   Std. Err.      z    P>|z|     [95% Conf. Interval]
-------------+----------------------------------------------------------------
intervention | -.1432429   .0649198    -2.21   0.027    -.2704833   -.0160025
    baseline |  .5243874   .0901241     5.82   0.000     .3477474    .7010275
       _cons | 1.356904    .2994742     4.53   0.000     .7699457   1.943863
------------------------------------------------------------------------------
```

Output 3.4   Results of the longitudinal GEE analysis of covariance

times the standard error. It can further be seen that the difference between the groups (i.e., the effect of the intervention) is adjusted for the differences between the groups at baseline, i.e., the baseline value is added to the model as a covariate. The last part of the output contains the random part of the model, which contains the random intercept variance (0.1129856). This variance indicates the variation between the subjects in the outcome variable or in other words, the amount of variance in the outcome explained by the differences between the subjects.

Output 3.4 shows the results of exactly the same analysis but now performed with a linear GEE analysis. In this GEE analysis, an exchangeable correlation structure is used.

The output of a longitudinal GEE analysis of covariance contains two parts, which are more or less the same as the first two parts of the output of the longitudinal mixed model analysis of covariance. In the first part, some general information is provided. This general information contains the group variable (id) and what kind of regression model is performed. In this situation a linear regression model is used (i.e., the link function is identity and the family is Gaussian). The information also shows that an exchangeable correlation structure is used for the estimation and it provides the scale parameter, which is a measure for the remaining unexplained variance after the analysis is performed. In the right column of the first part of the output, the same information is provided as has been provided in the first part of the output of the longitudinal mixed model analysis of covariance.

The second part of the output of a longitudinal GEE analysis of covariance provides the regression coefficients. The interpretation of the regression coefficient for the intervention variable (-0.1432429) is exactly the same as the interpretation of the regression coefficient of the intervention variable obtained from the longitudinal mixed model analysis of covariance. It also provides the standard error of the estimate (0.0649198), which is used in the calculation of the 95% confidence interval around the estimate, which ranges from -0.2704833 to -0.0160025 and the corresponding p-value (0.027). It should be noted that the effect estimate obtained from the longitudinal GEE analysis of covariance is almost the same as the one obtained from the longitudinal mixed model analysis of covariance (-0.1432429

versus -0.1419588). This is always the case. In fact, when there are no missing data, the regression coefficient obtained from a linear mixed model analysis with a random intercept is exactly the same as the regression coefficient obtained from a linear GEE analysis with an exchangeable correlation structure. This is caused by the fact that estimating one variance (the random intercept variance) is exactly the same as estimating one correlation (an exchangeable correlation structure) (Twisk, 2013). The only difference between the two regression coefficients in the present example is caused by missing data, and it is generally accepted that mixed model analysis deals better with missing data then GEE analysis (Twisk et al., 2013). Because the two methods to estimate the effect of the intervention almost give the same results and the fact that mixed models deals better with missing data, in the remaining part of this book, all examples with a continuous outcome variable will be analyzed with linear mixed model analyses.

After estimating the overall effect of the intervention on average over time, in a second step, the effects of the intervention at the (three) follow-up measurements can be estimated. With the longitudinal analysis of covariance, this is not done with three separate linear regression analyses, but this is done in one model. To assess the effect of the intervention at the different follow-up measurements, time and the interaction between the intervention variable and time are added to the model (Eq. 3.2):

$$Y_t = \beta_0 + \beta_1 X + \beta_2 Y_{t0} + \beta_3 time_2 + \beta_4 time_3 + \beta_5 X \times time_2 + \beta_6 X \times time_3 \quad (3.2)$$

where Y_t = outcome measured at the follow-up measurements, X = intervention variable, β_1 = intervention effect at the first follow-up measurement, Y_{t0} = outcome measured at baseline, and $time_2$, $time_3$ = dummy variables for the second and third follow-up measurement.

In this model, the regression coefficient for the intervention variable indicates the intervention effect at the first follow-up measurement. The intervention effect at the second follow-up measurement is calculated as the sum of the regression coefficient for the intervention variable and the regression coefficient for the interaction between the intervention variable and the time dummy variable for the second follow-up measurement ($\beta_1 + \beta_5$), while the intervention effect at the third follow-up measurement is calculated as the sum of the regression coefficient for the intervention variable and the regression coefficient for the interaction between the intervention variable and the time dummy variable for the third follow-up measurement ($\beta_1 + \beta_6$). Output 3.5 shows the result of this analysis.

Output 3.5 also contains three parts: the upper part which contains the overall information, the middle part which contains the fixed part of the model, and the lower part which contains the random part of the model. Most interesting is, of course, the middle part, because that part contains the regression coefficients. The analysis performed leads to a regression coefficient for the intervention variable, two regression coefficients for the time dummy variables, two regression coefficients for the interactions between the intervention variable and the two time dummy variables, and the regression coefficient for the baseline value. The latter indicates again that a longitudinal analysis of covariance was performed with an adjustment for the

```
Mixed-effects ML regression              Number of obs      =        416
Group variable: id                       Number of groups   =        150

                                         Obs per group:
                                                       min =          1
                                                       avg =        2.8
                                                       max =          3

                                         Wald chi2(6)       =      79.50
Log likelihood = -213.66378              Prob > chi2        =     0.0000

----------------------------------------------------------------------------
complaints |    Coef.   Std. Err.      z    P>|z|   [95% Conf. Interval]
-----------+----------------------------------------------------------------
intervention | -.1036192  .0785095   -1.32   0.187   -.2574949    .0502566
             |
       time  |
          2  | -.0826913  .0527159   -1.57   0.117   -.1860126    .0206301
          3  | -.1254292  .0530484   -2.36   0.018   -.2294022   -.0214562
             |
      time#  |
         c.  |
intervention |
          2  |  -.040448  .0763355   -0.53   0.596   -.1900627    .1091668
          3  | -.0799769  .0760742   -1.05   0.293   -.2290796    .0691258
             |
    baseline |  .5289271  .0778606    6.79   0.000    .3763233    .681531
       _cons | 1.410858   .2746856    5.14   0.000    .8724839   1.949232
----------------------------------------------------------------------------


----------------------------------------------------------------------------
Random-effects Parameters  |  Estimate  Std. Err.    [95% Conf. Interval]
---------------------------+------------------------------------------------
id: Identity               |
              var(_cons)   |  .1138685  .0179887     .0835474    .1551939
---------------------------+------------------------------------------------
            var(Residual)  |  .0978093  .0085373     .0824295    .1160587
----------------------------------------------------------------------------
LR test vs. linear model: chibar2(01) = 100.99      Prob >= chibar2 = 0.0000
```

Output 3.5 Results of the longitudinal mixed model analysis of covariance including an interaction between intervention and time

baseline value. The regression coefficient for the intervention variable (-0.1036192) indicates the difference between the intervention group and the control group at the first follow-up measurement (i.e., the reference time point). The regression coefficients for the two time dummy variables indicate the difference in complaints between the reference time point (i.e., the first follow-up measurement) and the other two follow-up measurements for the control group. These coefficients are, therefore, not really interesting. The regression coefficients for the two interactions terms indicate the difference between the first follow-up measurement and the other two follow-up measurements in the difference between the two groups. With these coefficients the effect estimates for the intervention at the second and third follow-up measurement can be calculated. For the second follow-up measurement, the effect estimate is $-0.1036192 + -0.040448 = -0.1440672$, while the effect estimate at the third follow-up measurement equals $-0.1036192 + -0.0799769 = -0.1835961$. The problem, however, is that although the effect estimates at the second and the third follow-up measurement can be calculated in this way, the standard errors (and therefore also the 95% confidence intervals and corresponding p-values) cannot be

```
Mixed-effects ML regression              Number of obs      =       416
Group variable: id                       Number of groups   =       150

                                         Obs per group:
                                                       min =         1
                                                       avg =       2.8
                                                       max =         3

                                         Wald chi2(6)       =     79.50
Log likelihood = -213.66378              Prob > chi2        =    0.0000

------------------------------------------------------------------------------
  complaints |     Coef.   Std. Err.      z    P>|z|    [95% Conf. Interval]
-------------+----------------------------------------------------------------
intervention | -.1440671   .0789085    -1.83   0.068    -.2987249    .0105907
             |
        time |
           1 |  .0826913   .0527159     1.57   0.117    -.0206301    .1860126
           3 | -.042738    .0525457    -0.81   0.416    -.1457256    .0602497
             |
       time# |
         c.  |
intervention |
           1 |  .040448    .0763355     0.53   0.596    -.1091668    .1900627
           3 | -.0395289   .076004     -0.52   0.603    -.188494     .1094361
             |
    baseline |  .5289271   .0778606     6.79   0.000     .3763233    .681531
       _cons |  1.328167   .2740424     4.85   0.000     .7910532   1.86528
------------------------------------------------------------------------------


------------------------------------------------------------------------------
  Random-effects Parameters  |   Estimate  Std. Err.    [95% Conf. Interval]
-----------------------------+------------------------------------------------
id: Identity                 |
                var(_cons)   |   .1138685   .0179887     .0835474    .1551939
-----------------------------+------------------------------------------------
                var(Residual)|   .0978093   .0085373     .0824295    .1160587
------------------------------------------------------------------------------
LR test vs. linear model: chibar2(01) = 100.99          Prob >= chibar2 = 0.0000
```

Output 3.6 Results of the longitudinal mixed model analysis of covariance including an interaction between intervention and time, with the second follow-up measurement as reference time point

calculated. To obtain these standard errors, the performed longitudinal analysis of covariance should be reanalyzed with a different reference category for time. Output 3.6. shows the result of the analysis with the second follow-up measurement as reference time point, and Output 3.7 shows the result of the analysis with the third follow-up measurement as reference time point.

From Output 3.6, it can be seen that the regression coefficient for the intervention variable equals -0.1440672, which is equal to the number calculated based on the two regression coefficients provided in Output 3.5. Besides the effect estimate, the output also gives the standard error of the estimate and, therefore, also the 95% confidence interval around the effect estimate and the corresponding p-value. In Output 3.7, the effect estimate at the third follow-up measurement is provided (0.1835961) with its 95% confidence interval and corresponding p-value.

```
Mixed-effects ML regression              Number of obs     =        416
Group variable: id                       Number of groups  =        150

                                         Obs per group:
                                                      min =          1
                                                      avg =        2.8
                                                      max =          3

                                         Wald chi2(6)      =      79.50
Log likelihood = -213.66378              Prob > chi2       =     0.0000

----------------------------------------------------------------------------
 complaints |    Coef.   Std. Err.     z    P>|z|    [95% Conf. Interval]
------------+---------------------------------------------------------------
intervention| -.1835961  .0783288   -2.34   0.019   -.3371176   -.0300745
            |
       time |
          1 |  .1254292  .0530484    2.36   0.018    .0214562    .2294022
          2 |   .042738  .0525457    0.81   0.416   -.0602497    .1457256
            |
      time#|
         c. |
intervention|
          1 |  .0799769  .0760742    1.05   0.293   -.0691258    .2290796
          2 |  .0395289   .076004    0.52   0.603   -.1094361    .188494
            |
   baseline |  .5289271  .0778606    6.79   0.000    .3763233    .681531
      _cons |  1.285429  .2749108    4.68   0.000    .7466132   1.824244
----------------------------------------------------------------------------


----------------------------------------------------------------------------
  Random-effects Parameters  |   Estimate   Std. Err.   [95% Conf. Interval]
-----------------------------+----------------------------------------------
Id: Identity                 |
                var(_cons)   |   .1138685   .0179887    .0835474    .1551939
-----------------------------+----------------------------------------------
              var(Residual)  |   .0978093   .0085373    .0824295    .1160587
----------------------------------------------------------------------------
LR test vs. linear model: chibar2(01) = 100.99    Prob >= chibar2 = 0.0000
```

Output 3.7 Results of the longitudinal mixed model analysis of covariance including an interaction between intervention and time, with the third follow-up measurement as reference time point

3.4.2 Repeated Measures

In the repeated measures analysis, the values of all four measurements of the outcome variable (i.e., the baseline value as well as the values of the three follow-up measurements) are used as outcome in the analysis. When the overall intervention effect is estimated, the model does not include time (Eq. 3.3), while when the intervention effect at the different follow-up measurements is estimated, time is represented by dummy variables (Eq. 3.4) . Because all four measurements are used as outcome, in the latter, three dummy variables are needed to represent time. The model includes further the interaction between intervention and time:

$$Y_t = \beta_0 + \beta_1 X \qquad (3.3)$$

where Y_t = outcome measured at all measurements, X = intervention variable, and β_1 = overall intervention effect.

Table 3.4 Data structure needed to perform a repeated measures analysis

Id	Outcome	Time	Intervention	Baseline
1	Y_{t0}	0	1	Na
1	Y_{t1}	1	1	Na
1	Y_{t2}	2	1	Na
1	Y_{t3}	3	1	Na

Na, not applicable

$$Y_t = \beta_0 + \beta_1 X + \beta_2 time_1 + \beta_3 time_2 + \beta_4 time_3 + \beta_5 X \times time_1 + \beta_6 X \\ \times time_2 + \beta_7 X \times time_3 X + \beta_2 time_1 + \beta_3 time_2 + \beta_4 time_3 + \beta_5 X \\ \times time_1 + \beta_6 X \times time_2 + \beta_7 X \times time_3 \tag{3.4}$$

where Y_t = outcome measured at all measurements, X = intervention variable, β_1 = difference between the groups at baseline, and $time_2$, $time_3$, $time_4$ = dummy variables for the first, second, and third follow-up measurement.

Table 3.4 shows the structure of the data used to estimate the parameters of a repeated measures analysis.

In Eq. 3.3, the regression coefficient for the treatment variable indicates the difference between the intervention and control groups on average over time. In the model with the three dummy variables (Eq. 3.4), the intervention effect at the first follow-up measurement is calculated as the sum of the regression coefficient for the intervention variable and the regression coefficient for the interaction between the intervention variable and the dummy variable for the first follow-up measurement ($\beta_1 + \beta_5$), while the intervention effect at the second follow-up measurement is calculated as the sum of the regression coefficient for the intervention variable and the regression coefficient for the interaction between the intervention variable and the dummy variable for the second follow-up measurement ($\beta_1 + \beta_6$). And of course, the intervention effect at the third follow-up measurement is calculated as the sum of the regression coefficient for the intervention variable and the regression coefficient for the interaction between the intervention variable and the dummy variable for the third follow-up measurement ($\beta_1 + \beta_7$).

In the repeated measures analysis, the baseline value is part of the outcome (see Table 3.4), and therefore it is not possible to adjust for the baseline values as well. Although some researchers try to do so, it does not make sense, because in that situation the baseline value as outcome is adjusted for itself. So, therefore, the analysis is relatively simple and only contains the intervention variable (Eq. 3.3). Output 3.8 shows the result of the analysis.

In the upper part of Output 3.8, it can be seen that the maximal number of measurements for each subject is equal to 4, which shows that in this analysis, the baseline value is part of the outcome. As for the outputs of the longitudinal analysis of covariance, the most interesting part of the output is the middle part which contains the effect estimate for the intervention. The effect estimate is the regression coefficient for the intervention variable (-0.2480394), which indicates the difference between the intervention and control groups on average over time. It should be realized that this effect estimate includes the difference between the two groups at baseline, which is not caused by the intervention.

```
Mixed-effects ML regression                    Number of obs      =        572
Group variable: id                             Number of groups   =        156

                                               Obs per group:
                                                            min =          1
                                                            avg =        3.7
                                                            max =          4

                                               Wald chi2(1)       =      15.55
Log likelihood = -359.90801                    Prob > chi2        =     0.0001

------------------------------------------------------------------------------
  complaints |     Coef.   Std. Err.      z    P>|z|    [95% Conf. Interval]
-------------+----------------------------------------------------------------
intervention | -.2480394   .0629007    -3.94   0.000   -.3713225   -.1247562
       _cons |  3.262652   .0433469    75.27   0.000    3.177694    3.34761
------------------------------------------------------------------------------


------------------------------------------------------------------------------
Random-effects Parameters  |   Estimate   Std. Err.    [95% Conf. Interval]
---------------------------+--------------------------------------------------
id: Identity               |
                var(_cons) |   .1127726   .0176065     .0830445    .1531427
---------------------------+--------------------------------------------------
             var(Residual) |   .1428889   .0098981     .1247483    .1636676
------------------------------------------------------------------------------
LR test vs. linear model: chibar2(01) = 122.69     Prob >= chibar2 = 0.0000
```

Output 3.8 Results of the longitudinal repeated measures mixed model analysis

With the repeated measures analysis, it is also possible to obtain the effects of the intervention at the different time points. Therefore, three time dummy variables and the interaction between the intervention variable and the three time dummy variables were added to the model (Eq. 3.3). Although the default option in analyses with a categorical variable (i.e., time) is to take the first category as reference category, in this particular situation that makes no sense. Because the first category indicates the first measurement (i.e., the baseline value), the estimated difference between the groups at the first measurement is not related to the intervention and, therefore, not an actual effect estimate of the intervention. Therefore, in the first analysis, the second measurement (i.e., the first follow-up measurement) is used as reference category. Output 3.9 shows the results of this analysis.

It has been mentioned before that from Output 3.9, the most interesting regression coefficient is the coefficient for the intervention variable (-0.2212681). That coefficient indicates the difference between the intervention and control groups at the first follow-up measurement. It has also been mentioned before that the regression coefficients given in Output 3.9 can also be used to calculate the effect estimates for the intervention at the second and third follow-up measurement. To do so, the regression coefficient of the intervention variable has to be added to the regression coefficients of the interactions between the intervention variable and the corresponding time dummy variable. So, the effect estimate for the intervention at the second follow-up measurement equals $-0.2212681 + -0.0502898 = -0.2715579$, while the effect estimate for the intervention at the third follow-up measurement equals $-0.2212681 + -0.0774314 = -0.2986995$. The problem of these calculations is (again) that there is no estimation of the standard errors of the estimates, and therefore there is no estimation of the 95% confidence intervals and

```
Mixed-effects ML regression                     Number of obs      =       572
Group variable: id                              Number of groups   =       156

                                                Obs per group:
                                                             min =         1
                                                             avg =       3.7
                                                             max =         4

                                                Wald chi2(7)       =    131.78
Log likelihood = -308.62968                     Prob > chi2        =    0.0000

-----------------------------------------------------------------------------
  complaints |     Coef.   Std. Err.      z    P>|z|    [95% Conf. Interval]
-------------+---------------------------------------------------------------
intervention |  -.2212681   .0803815    -2.75  0.006   -.378813    -.0637231
             |
        time |
           1 |   .2199861   .0548916     4.01  0.000    .1124005    .3275718
           3 |  -.0785976   .0561745    -1.40  0.162   -.1886976    .0315024
           4 |  -.1314942   .0564121    -2.33  0.020   -.2420599   -.0209284
             |
       time#|
          c. |
intervention |
           1 |    .006242   .078879      0.08  0.937   -.148358     .160842
           3 |  -.0502898   .0813001    -0.62  0.536   -.2096351    .1090554
           4 |  -.0774314   .0809424    -0.96  0.339   -.2360755    .0812128
             |
       _cons |   3.249611   .0559161    58.12  0.000    3.140017    3.359204
-----------------------------------------------------------------------------


-----------------------------------------------------------------------------
  Random-effects Parameters |   Estimate   Std. Err.     [95% Conf. Interval]
----------------------------+------------------------------------------------
id: Identity                |
              var(_cons)    |   .1211421   .0175331      .0912219    .1608759
----------------------------+------------------------------------------------
             var(Residual)  |    .111834   .0077539      .097624     .1281123
-----------------------------------------------------------------------------
LR test vs. linear model: chibar2(01) = 171.28       Prob >= chibar2 = 0.0000
```

Output 3.9 Results of the longitudinal mixed model repeated measures analysis including an interaction between intervention and time, with the second measurement (i.e., the first follow-up measurement) as reference time point

the corresponding *p*-values. To obtain those, the repeated measures analysis with the interaction between the intervention variable and time must be performed with different reference categories for time. Outputs 3.10 and 3.11 show the results of the analyses with the second follow-up measurement and the third follow-up measurement as reference category.

The regression coefficient of the intervention variable provided by Output 3.10 (−0.2715579) gives the effect estimate for the intervention at the second follow-up, while the regression coefficient of the group variable provided by Output 3.11 (−0.2986994) gives the effect estimate for the intervention at the third follow-up. Although these effect estimates were already known from the calculation performed on the regression coefficients provided in Output 3.6, now for both effect estimates, also the standard errors are given, which are used in the estimation of the 95% confidence intervals and the corresponding *p*-values.

Although the repeated measures analyses performed so far included the baseline value, it should be noted again that in this analysis there is no adjustment for the

```
Mixed-effects ML regression                Number of obs     =        572
Group variable: id                         Number of groups  =        156

                                           Obs per group:
                                                          min =          1
                                                          avg =        3.7
                                                          max =          4

                                           Wald chi2(7)      =     131.78
Log likelihood = -308.62968                Prob > chi2       =     0.0000

------------------------------------------------------------------------------
 complaints |    Coef.   Std. Err.      z    P>|z|     [95% Conf. Interval]
------------+-----------------------------------------------------------------
intervention| -.2715579  .0808956   -3.36   0.001    -.4301104   -.1130054
            |
       time |
          1 |  .2985838  .0543956    5.49   0.000     .1919705    .4051971
          2 |  .0785976  .0561745    1.40   0.162    -.0315024    .1886976
          4 | -.0528965  .0559115   -0.95   0.344    -.162481     .0566879
            |
      time# |
         c. |
intervention|
          1 |  .0565318  .0794028    0.71   0.476    -.0990948    .2121584
          2 |  .0502898  .0813001    0.62   0.536    -.1090554    .2096351
          4 | -.0271415  .0810235   -0.33   0.738    -.1859447    .1316617
            |
       _cons|  3.171013  .0554291   57.21   0.000     3.062374    3.279652
------------------------------------------------------------------------------


------------------------------------------------------------------------------
  Random-effects Parameters  |  Estimate  Std. Err.    [95% Conf. Interval]
-----------------------------+------------------------------------------------
id: Identity                 |
                 var(_cons)  |  .1211421  .0175331     .0912219    .1608759
-----------------------------+------------------------------------------------
              var(Residual)  |  .111834   .0077539     .097624     .1281123
------------------------------------------------------------------------------
LR test vs. linear model: chibar2(01) = 171.28      Prob >= chibar2 = 0.0000
```

Output 3.10 Results of the longitudinal mixed model repeated measures analysis including an interaction between intervention and time, with the third measurement (i.e., the second follow-up measurement) as reference time point

baseline value. This is a general misunderstanding. Many researchers do believe that the repeated measures analysis performed does adjust for the baseline value. However, because the baseline value in these analyses is treated as an outcome instead of a covariate, the method actually does not adjust for the baseline value. To obtain an effect estimate of the intervention with a repeated measures analysis adjusted for the baseline, an alternative repeated measures analysis can be used. In this alternative repeated measures analysis, the intervention variable is not part of the model, but its interaction with time still is (Eqs. 3.5 and 3.6):

$$Y_t = \beta_0 + \beta_1 time + \beta_2 X \times time \qquad (3.5)$$

where Y_t = outcome measured at all measurements, X = intervention variable, and β_2 = overall intervention effect.

```
Mixed-effects ML regression                    Number of obs      =        572
Group variable: id                             Number of groups   =        156

                                               Obs per group:
                                                            min =          1
                                                            avg =        3.7
                                                            max =          4

                                               Wald chi2(7)       =     131.78
Log likelihood = -308.62968                    Prob > chi2        =     0.0000

------------------------------------------------------------------------------
 complaints |     Coef.   Std. Err.      z    P>|z|     [95% Conf. Interval]
------------+-----------------------------------------------------------------
intervention| -.2986994   .0802546   -3.72   0.000    -.4559956   -.1414033
            |
       time |
          1 |  .3514803    .054366    6.47   0.000     .2449249    .4580357
          2 |  .1314942   .0564121    2.33   0.020     .0209284    .2420599
          3 |  .0528965   .0559115    0.95   0.344    -.0566879    .162481
            |
      time#|
         c. |
intervention|
          1 |  .0836733   .0787496    1.06   0.288    -.0706731    .2380198
          2 |  .0774314   .0809424    0.96   0.339    -.0812128    .2360755
          3 |  .0271415   .0810235    0.33   0.738    -.1316617    .1859447
            |
      _cons |  3.118117   .0554001   56.28   0.000     3.009534    3.226699
------------------------------------------------------------------------------


------------------------------------------------------------------------------
  Random-effects Parameters  |   Estimate   Std. Err.     [95% Conf. Interval]
-----------------------------+------------------------------------------------
id: Identity                 |
                 var(_cons)  |   .1211421   .0175331      .0912219    .1608759
-----------------------------+------------------------------------------------
               var(Residual) |   .111834    .0077539      .097624     .1281123
------------------------------------------------------------------------------
LR test vs. linear model: chibar2(01) = 171.28         Prob >= chibar2 = 0.0000
```

Output 3.11 Results of the longitudinal mixed model repeated measures analysis including an interaction between intervention and time, with the fourth measurement (i.e., the third follow-up measurement) as reference time point

$$Y_t = \beta_0 + \beta_1 time_1 + \beta_2 time_2 + \beta_3 time_3 + \beta_4 X \times time_1 + \beta_5 X \times time_2$$
$$+ \beta_6 X \times time_3 \qquad (3.6)$$

where Y_t = outcome measured at all measurements, X = intervention variable, β_4 = intervention effect at the first follow-up measurement, β_5 = intervention effect at the second follow-up measurement, β_6 = intervention effect at the third follow-up measurement, and $time_1$, $time_2$, $time_3$ = dummy variables for the first, second, and third follow-up measurement.

Table 3.5 shows the structure of the data used to estimate the parameters of an alternative repeated measures analysis.

Because the intervention variable is not included in the model, the baseline values for both groups are assumed to be equal and are reflected in the intercept of the model (β_0). The intervention effects can be directly obtained from the regression coefficients for the interaction between the treatment variable and time (the overall treatment effect over time; β_2 in Eq. 3.5) or between the treatment variable and the

Table 3.5 Data structure needed to perform the alternative repeated measures analysis

Id	Outcome	Time1	Time2	Intervention	Baseline
1	Y_{t0}	0	0	1	Na
1	Y_{t1}	1	1	1	Na
1	Y_{t2}	1	2	1	Na
1	Y_{t3}	1	3	1	Na

Na, not applicable; Time1 = time variable needed to estimate the overall intervention effect; Time2 = time variable needed to estimate the intervention effects at the different follow-up measurements

three dummy variables for time (intervention effects at the three follow-up measurements: β_4, β_5, and β_6 in Eq. 3.7).

First, the alternative repeated measures mixed model analysis is applied to estimate the overall intervention effect on average over time. The model only includes time (coded 0 for the baseline value and 1 for all follow-up measurements; see Table 3.5) and the interaction between the intervention variable and time. Output 3.12 shows the result of this analysis.

From Output 3.12, the most important estimate is the regression coefficient for the interaction between the intervention variable and time (-0.1503951). This coefficient indicates the difference between the intervention and control groups on average over time. Because the intervention variable is not present in the model, the β_0 (3.367597) is an estimation of the outcome (i.e., complaints) for the whole population when the time variable equals 0, which is in this situation the baseline value (see Table 3.5). Because it is an estimation for the whole population, it implies that the baseline value is assumed to be equal for both groups, which implicates that the analysis is adjusted for the baseline value.

To get effect estimates of the intervention at the three follow-up measurements, for each follow-up measurement, a time dummy variable must be used, and for all these three dummy variables, an interaction with the intervention variable must be added to the model. Again, the intervention variable itself is not part of the model (see Eq. 3.6). Output 3.13 shows the results of this analysis.

The regression coefficients of interest from Output 3.13 are the three regression coefficients for the interactions between the intervention variable and the time dummy variables. These regression coefficients directly provide the effect estimates for the intervention at the three follow-up measurements. The regression coefficient for the interaction between the intervention variable and the dummy variable for the first follow-up measurement (-0.1077524) indicates the intervention effect at the first follow-up measurement, and the regression coefficient for the interaction between the intervention variable and the dummy variable for the second follow-up measurement (-0.1579727) indicates the intervention effect at the second follow-up measurement, while the regression coefficient for the interaction between the intervention variable and the dummy variable for the third follow-up measurement (-0.1852883) indicates the intervention effect at the third follow-up measurement. All these effect estimates are adjusted for the baseline value, because (again)

```
Mixed-effects ML regression                      Number of obs      =        572
Group variable: id                               Number of groups   =        156

                                                 Obs per group:
                                                            min =              1
                                                            avg =            3.7
                                                            max =              4

                                                 Wald chi2(2)       =     100.45
Log likelihood = -321.52225                      Prob > chi2        =     0.0000

------------------------------------------------------------------------------
 complaints |      Coef.   Std. Err.      z    P>|z|     [95% Conf. Interval]
------------+-----------------------------------------------------------------
       time |  -.2415208   .0411313    -5.87   0.000    -.3221366    -.160905
 inter_time |  -.1503951   .0528063    -2.85   0.004    -.2538936   -.0468966
       _cons |   3.367597   .0393959    85.48   0.000     3.290383    3.444812
------------------------------------------------------------------------------


------------------------------------------------------------------------------
 Random-effects Parameters  |   Estimate   Std. Err.     [95% Conf. Interval]
----------------------------+-------------------------------------------------
id: Identity                |
                 var(_cons) |   .1245786    .018348      .0933422     .166268
----------------------------+-------------------------------------------------
               var(Residual) |   .1175388   .0081834     .1025458     .134724
------------------------------------------------------------------------------
LR test vs. linear model: chibar2(01) = 162.12         Prob >= chibar2 = 0.0000
```

Output 3.12   Results of the alternative longitudinal mixed model repeated measures analysis

the intervention variable itself is not added to the model. A nice advantage of the analysis performed is that for all effect estimates at the different follow-up measurements, the corresponding standard errors are estimated directly, and, therefore, the 95% confidence intervals around the effect estimates and the corresponding p-values are directly provided by Output 3.13. So, it is not necessary to reanalyze the data with different reference categories for the different follow-up measurements.

3.4.3   Analysis of Changes

In the third method to analyze RCT data with more than one follow-up measurement, not the observed values at the different follow-up measurements are analyzed but the changes between the baseline measurement and the first follow-up measurement, between the baseline measurement and the second follow-up measurement, and between the baseline measurement and the third follow-up measurement (Eq. 3.7):

$$Y_t - Y_{t0} = \beta_0 + \beta_1 X \tag{3.7}$$

where Y_t = outcome measured at the follow-up measurements; Y_{t0}= outcome measured at baseline; X = intervention variable, and β_1 = overall intervention effect.

Although, it is sometimes suggested that the analysis of changes takes into account the difference between the groups at baseline, this is not the case (see

```
Mixed-effects ML regression                    Number of obs     =        572
Group variable: id                             Number of groups  =        156

                                               Obs per group:
                                                            min =          1
                                                            avg =        3.7
                                                            max =          4

                                               Wald chi2(6)      =     123.02
Log likelihood = -312.44411                    Prob > chi2       =     0.0000

------------------------------------------------------------------------------
 complaints |     Coef.   Std. Err.      z    P>|z|    [95% Conf. Interval]
------------+-----------------------------------------------------------------
   _Itime_2 |  -.1718823   .0522051    -3.29   0.001   -.2742024   -.0695623
   _Itime_3 |  -.2504772   .0516792    -4.85   0.000   -.3517665   -.1491879
   _Itime_4 |  -.3033201   .0516473    -5.87   0.000   -.4045469   -.2020933
  int_time2 |  -.1077524   .0699797    -1.54   0.124   -.2449101    .0294054
  int_time3 |  -.1579727   .0705751    -2.24   0.025   -.2962974    -.019648
  int_time4 |  -.1852883   .0698331    -2.65   0.008   -.3221587   -.0484179
      _cons |   3.367597   .0391056    86.12   0.000    3.290952    3.444243
------------------------------------------------------------------------------


------------------------------------------------------------------------------
  Random-effects Parameters  |   Estimate   Std. Err.    [95% Conf. Interval]
-----------------------------+------------------------------------------------
id: Identity                 |
                  var(_cons) |   .1260466   .0183463     .0947628    .1676582
-----------------------------+------------------------------------------------
               var(Residual) |   .1125164   .0078346     .0981626    .1289691
------------------------------------------------------------------------------
LR test vs. linear model: chibar2(01) = 171.33        Prob >= chibar2 = 0.0000
```

Output 3.13 Results of the alternative longitudinal mixed model repeated measures analysis including an interaction between intervention and time

Sect. 2.1), and, therefore, this method can also be performed with an adjustment for the baseline value of the outcome variable (Eq. 3.8):

$$Y_t - Y_{t0} = \beta_0 + \beta_1 X + \beta_2 Y_{t0} \qquad (3.8)$$

where Y_t = outcome measured at the follow-up measurements, Y_{t0}= outcome measured at baseline, X = intervention variable, and β_1= overall intervention effect.

As in all other discussed methods, the model can be extended with time and the interaction between the intervention variable and time to estimate the effect of the intervention at the different follow-up measurements (Eqs. 3.9 and 3.10):

$$Y_t - Y_{t0} = \beta_0 + \beta_1 X + \beta_2 time_2 + + \beta_3 time_3 + \beta_4 X \times time_2 + + \beta_5 X \\ \times time_3 \qquad (3.9)$$

$$Y_t - Y_{t0} = \beta_0 + \beta_1 X + \beta_2 Y_{t0} + \beta_3 time_2 + \beta_4 time_3 + \beta_5 X \times time_2 + \beta_6 X \\ \times time_3 \qquad (3.10)$$

where Y_t = outcome measured at the follow-up measurements, Y_{t0}=outcome measured at baseline, X = intervention variable, β_1= intervention effect at the first follow-up measurement, and $time_2$, $time_3$ = dummy variables for the second and third follow-up measurement.

Table 3.6 Data structure needed to perform an analysis of changes

id	Outcome	Time	Intervention	Baseline
1	$Y_{t1} - Y_{t0}$	0	1	Y_{t0}
1	$Y_{t2} - Y_{t0}$	1	1	Y_{t0}
1	$Y_{t3} - Y_{t0}$	2	1	Y_{t0}

The overall intervention effect and the intervention effects at the three follow-up measurements can be obtained in the same way as been described for the longitudinal analysis of covariance (see Sect. 3.4.1). Table 3.6 shows the structure of the data used to estimate the parameters of the analysis of changes.

Output 3.14 shows the result of the mixed model analysis performed on the change scores in the outcome variable. The three change scores are calculated as the difference between the baseline value and the three follow-up measurements (see Eq. 3.7 and Table 3.6).

The output of the longitudinal mixed model analysis of changes looks similar to the outputs of the mixed model analyses performed earlier. From the first part of Output 3.14, it can be seen that there are a maximum number of three observations: i.e., the three change scores between the baseline measurement and the three follow-up measurements. In the second part of the output (the fixed part of the model), the regression coefficients are given. The regression coefficient for the intervention variable (-0.0522368) indicates the overall intervention effect on average over time. This intervention effect actually is the difference between the groups in the changes between the baseline measurement and the three follow-up measurements. In Chap. 2 it was already argued that analyzing change scores (can) lead to bias in the effect estimates due to regression to the mean. It was also argued that a solution to this problem is to adjust the analysis of the change score for the baseline value. It has been mentioned before that this solution can also be applied for the longitudinal analysis of change scores (see Eq. 3.8). Output 3.15 shows the result of the analysis.

In the middle part of Output 3.15 (the fixed part of the model), it can be seen that an adjustment is made for the baseline value of the outcome variable. The regression coefficient of the intervention variable (-0.1419588) again indicates the overall intervention effect on average over time, i.e., the difference between the groups in the differences between the baseline value and the three follow-up measurements. This difference, however, is now adjusted for the baseline differences between the groups.

In the same way, it is of course also possible to obtain the effects of the intervention at the different follow-up measurements. Therefore, the models have to be extended with time (i.e., two time dummy variables) and the interaction between the intervention variable and time (see Eqs. 3.9 and 3.10). Output 3.16 and 3.17 show the results of the two analyses. In the first analysis, there is no adjustment for the baseline value, while in the second analysis, the baseline value of the outcome is added to the model.

As has been mentioned before, in Outputs 3.16 and 3.17, the regression coefficient for the intervention variable indicates the effect of the intervention at the

```
Mixed-effects ML regression                    Number of obs      =        416
Group variable: id                             Number of groups   =        150

                                               Obs per group:
                                                            min =          1
                                                            avg =        2.8
                                                            max =          3

                                               Wald chi2(1)       =       0.53
Log likelihood = -239.86042                    Prob > chi2        =     0.4655

---------------------------------------------------------------------------------
 change_com |    Coef.    Std. Err.     z    P>|z|    [95% Conf. Interval]
------------+--------------------------------------------------------------------
intervention| -.0522368    .07158    -0.73   0.466    -.1925311    .0880575
      _cons | -.2897832   .0493003    -5.88   0.000    -.3864101   -.1931563
---------------------------------------------------------------------------------


---------------------------------------------------------------------------------
 Random-effects Parameters  |   Estimate   Std. Err.    [95% Conf. Interval]
----------------------------+----------------------------------------------------
id: Identity                |
              var(_cons)    |   .1519201   .0226676      .113399    .2035265
----------------------------+----------------------------------------------------
            var(Residual)   |   .1041805   .0090848     .0878131    .1235986
---------------------------------------------------------------------------------
LR test vs. linear model: chibar2(01) = 125.80       Prob >= chibar2 = 0.0000
```

Output 3.14 Results of the longitudinal mixed model analysis of changes

```
Mixed-effects ML regression                    Number of obs      =        416
Group variable: id                             Number of groups   =        150

                                               Obs per group:
                                                            min =          1
                                                            avg =        2.8
                                                            max =          3

                                               Wald chi2(2)       =      37.66
Log likelihood = -223.41988                    Prob > chi2        =     0.0000

---------------------------------------------------------------------------------
 change_com |    Coef.    Std. Err.     z    P>|z|    [95% Conf. Interval]
------------+--------------------------------------------------------------------
intervention| -.1419588   .0654837    -2.17   0.030    -.2703044   -.0136132
   baseline | -.4756309   .0782574    -6.08   0.000    -.6290127   -.3222491
      _cons |  1.356396   .2742621     4.95   0.000     .818852     1.89394
---------------------------------------------------------------------------------


---------------------------------------------------------------------------------
 Random-effects Parameters  |   Estimate   Std. Err.    [95% Conf. Interval]
----------------------------+----------------------------------------------------
 id: Identity               |
              var(_cons)    |   .1129856   .0182538     .0823197    .1550753
----------------------------+----------------------------------------------------
            var(Residual)   |    .104595   .0091373     .0881356    .1241282
---------------------------------------------------------------------------------
LR test vs. linear model: chibar2(01) = 92.75        Prob >= chibar2 = 0.0000
```

Output 3.15 Results of the longitudinal mixed model analysis of changes adjusted for the baseline value

```
Mixed-effects ML regression                  Number of obs      =        416
Group variable: id                           Number of groups   =        150

                                             Obs per group:
                                                          min =          1
                                                          avg =        2.8
                                                          max =          3

                                             Wald chi2(5)       =      20.92
Log likelihood = -229.97356                  Prob > chi2        =     0.0008

------------------------------------------------------------------------------
  change_com |      Coef.   Std. Err.      z    P>|z|     [95% Conf. Interval]
-------------+----------------------------------------------------------------
intervention |  -.0139447   .0834508    -0.17   0.867    -.1775052    .1496158
             |
        time |
           2 |  -.0811427   .0526752    -1.54   0.123    -.1843843    .0220988
           3 |  -.1248979   .0530481    -2.35   0.019    -.2288703   -.0209256
             |
       time# |
          c. |
intervention |
           2 |   -.041143   .0762928    -0.54   0.590    -.1906742    .1083881
           3 |  -.0830853   .0760637    -1.09   0.275    -.2321674    .0659969
             |
       _cons |  -.2200715   .0579953    -3.79   0.000    -.3337402   -.1064028
------------------------------------------------------------------------------


------------------------------------------------------------------------------
  Random-effects Parameters  |   Estimate   Std. Err.    [95% Conf. Interval]
-----------------------------+------------------------------------------------
id: Identity                 |
                 var(_cons)  |   .1519348   .0223081     .1139405    .2025987
-----------------------------+------------------------------------------------
              var(Residual)  |   .0974508   .0084917     .0821511    .1155999
------------------------------------------------------------------------------
LR test vs. linear model: chibar2(01) = 134.92        Prob >= chibar2 = 0.0000
```

Output 3.16 Results of the longitudinal mixed model analysis of changes including an interaction between intervention and time

reference time point, which is the first follow-up measurement. Without an adjustment for the baseline value, the intervention effect at the first follow-up measurement equals -0.0139447, while with an adjustment for the baseline value, the effect estimate equals -0.1036192. The difference illustrates nicely the importance of the adjustment for the baseline value, i.e., the adjustment for the baseline differences between the two groups.

As for all analyses with an interaction term, based on the analyses performed, it is possible to calculate the effect estimates at the other two follow-up measurements. Therefore, the regression coefficient for the interaction between the particular time dummy variable and the intervention variable has to be added to the regression coefficient for the intervention variable itself. For instance, the intervention effect at the second follow-up measurement based on the analysis of changes with an adjustment for the baseline value (Output 3.17) equals $-0.1036192 + -0.040448 = -0.1440672$. Although Outputs 3.16 and 3.17 can be used to calculate the effect estimates at the different time points, they cannot be used to calculate the standard errors of these estimates, and therefore they can also

```
Mixed-effects ML regression              Number of obs     =        416
Group variable: id                       Number of groups  =        150

                                         Obs per group:
                                                        min =          1
                                                        avg =        2.8
                                                        max =          3

                                         Wald chi2(6)      =      58.18
Log likelihood = -213.66378              Prob > chi2       =     0.0000

--------------------------------------------------------------------------------
  change_com |    Coef.   Std. Err.      z    P>|z|    [95% Conf. Interval]
-------------+------------------------------------------------------------------
intervention | -.1036192   .0785095   -1.32   0.187   -.2574949     .0502566
             |
        time |
           2 | -.0826913   .0527159   -1.57   0.117   -.1860126     .0206301
           3 | -.1254292   .0530484   -2.36   0.018   -.2294022    -.0214562
             |
       time# |
          c. |
intervention |
           2 |  -.040448   .0763355   -0.53   0.596   -.1900627     .1091668
           3 | -.0799769   .0760742   -1.05   0.293   -.2290796     .0691258
             |
    baseline | -.4710729   .0778606   -6.05   0.000   -.6236767    -.318469
       _cons |  1.410858   .2746856    5.14   0.000    .8724839    1.949232
--------------------------------------------------------------------------------


--------------------------------------------------------------------------------
  Random-effects Parameters  |   Estimate   Std. Err.    [95% Conf. Interval]
-----------------------------+--------------------------------------------------
id: Identity                 |
                var(_cons)   |   .1138685   .0179887      .0835474     .1551939
-----------------------------+--------------------------------------------------
             var(Residual)   |   .0978093   .0085373      .0824295     .1160587
--------------------------------------------------------------------------------
LR test vs. linear model: chibar2(01) = 100.99       Prob >= chibar2 = 0.0000
```

Output 3.17 Results of the longitudinal mixed model analysis of changes including an interaction between intervention and time, adjusted for the baseline value

not be used to calculate the 95% confidence intervals around the effect estimates and the corresponding p-values. To obtain the 95% confidence intervals and p-values, the analyses have to be redone with different reference categories for the time dummy variables. Outputs 3.18–3.21 show the results of these analyses, both without and with an adjustment for the baseline value.

3.5   Overview and Discussion

Table 3.7 shows an overview of the results obtained from the different analyses in order to estimate the overall intervention effect on average over time, while Table 3.8 shows an overview of the results obtained from the different analyses in order to estimate the effect of the intervention at the different follow-up measurements.

From Tables 3.7 and 3.8, it is obvious that the effect estimates differ remarkably between the different methods used to estimate the effect of an RCT with more than

```
Mixed-effects ML regression                    Number of obs      =        416
Group variable: id                             Number of groups   =        150

                                               Obs per group:
                                                          min =          1
                                                          avg =        2.8
                                                          max =          3

                                               Wald chi2(5)       =      20.92
Log likelihood = -229.97356                    Prob > chi2        =     0.0008

----------------------------------------------------------------------------------
  change_com |      Coef.    Std. Err.      z     P>|z|     [95% Conf. Interval]
-------------+--------------------------------------------------------------------
intervention |   -.0550877    .0839889    -0.66    0.512    -.2197029     .1095274
             |
        time |
           1 |    .0811427    .0526752     1.54    0.123    -.0220988     .1843843
           3 |   -.0437552     .052527    -0.83    0.405    -.1467062     .0591958
             |
       time# |
          c. |
intervention |
           1 |    .041143     .0762928     0.54    0.590    -.1083881     .1906742
           3 |   -.0419422    .0759417    -0.55    0.581    -.1907853     .1069008
             |
       _cons |   -.3012142    .0575453    -5.23    0.000     -.414001    -.1884275
----------------------------------------------------------------------------------


----------------------------------------------------------------------------------
  Random-effects Parameters  |   Estimate   Std. Err.    [95% Conf. Interval]
-----------------------------+----------------------------------------------------
id: Identity                 |
                 var(_cons)  |   .1519348   .0223081      .1139405     .2025987
-----------------------------+----------------------------------------------------
              var(Residual)  |   .0974508   .0084917      .0821511     .1155999
----------------------------------------------------------------------------------
LR test vs. linear model: chibar2(01) = 134.92          Prob >= chibar2 = 0.0000
```

Output 3.18 Results of the longitudinal mixed model analysis of changes including an interaction between intervention and time with the second follow-up measurement as reference time point

one follow-up measurement. This is partly caused by the observed differences at baseline between the groups. In Table 3.1 it could be seen that the baseline value for the intervention group was lower than the baseline value for the control group (3.25 for the intervention group and 3.47 for the control group). Because of that, the decrease over time in the intervention group is (much) harder to achieve than the decrease over time in the control group. The control group tends to decrease over time due to regression to the mean, while the intervention group tends to increase over time due to regression to the mean. Because of that the analysis of changes without adjustment for the baseline leads to an underestimation of the intervention effects. The repeated measure analyses on the other hand lead to an overestimation of the effect estimates. In these analyses the differences between the groups at baseline are part of the estimated differences between the groups, i.e., are part of the effect estimates. Because the baseline differences between the groups are in favor of the intervention group (the intervention group has a lower complaint score at baseline than the control group), the effect estimates, which include the baseline difference, are (highly) overestimated.

```
Mixed-effects ML regression                    Number of obs      =        416
Group variable: id                             Number of groups   =        150

                                               Obs per group:
                                                           min =          1
                                                           avg =        2.8
                                                           max =          3

                                               Wald chi2(5)       =      20.92
Log likelihood = -229.97356                    Prob > chi2        =     0.0008

-----------------------------------------------------------------------------
 change_com |    Coef.   Std. Err.      z    P>|z|     [95% Conf. Interval]
------------+----------------------------------------------------------------
intervention |   -.09703   .083358   -1.16   0.244   -.2604086    .0663487
             |
        time |
           1 |  .1248979  .0530481    2.35   0.019    .0209256    .2288703
           2 |  .0437552   .052527    0.83   0.405   -.0591958    .1467062
             |
       time# |
          c. |
intervention |
           1 |  .0830853  .0760637    1.09   0.275   -.0659969    .2321674
           2 |  .0419422  .0759417    0.55   0.581   -.1069008    .1907853
             |
       _cons |  -.3449694  .0574813   -6.00   0.000   -.4576307   -.2323082
-----------------------------------------------------------------------------


-----------------------------------------------------------------------------
 Random-effects Parameters  |  Estimate   Std. Err.    [95% Conf. Interval]
----------------------------+------------------------------------------------
id: Identity                |
               var(_cons)   |  .1519348   .0223081     .1139405    .2025987
----------------------------+------------------------------------------------
            var(Residual)   |  .0974508   .0084917     .0821511    .1155999
-----------------------------------------------------------------------------
LR test vs. linear model: chibar2(01) = 134.92      Prob >= chibar2 = 0.0000
```

Output 3.19 Results of the longitudinal mixed model analysis of changes including an interaction between intervention and time with the third follow-up measurement as reference time point

It was already mentioned in Chap. 2 that regarding the adjustment for the baseline value, it does not matter whether the outcome variable is the observed value at the different follow-up measurements (i.e., longitudinal analysis of covariance) or the changes between the baseline measurement and the follow-up measurements (i.e., analysis of changes); the effect estimates are exactly the same in both methods. The mathematical equivalence between the two methods leading to the same estimation of the treatment effect was already explained in Chap. 2 (see Box 2.1).

Although the general idea is the same, the results of the alternative repeated measures analysis without the treatment variable in the model (Eqs. 3.4 and 3.5) slightly differed from the results of the longitudinal analysis of covariance. The advantage of the alternative repeated measures analysis is that also subjects with only a baseline measurement are included in the analysis. So, in the present example, the two analyses are based on a slightly different population. However, also when the method is used in a dataset without any missing data, the results of the alternative repeated measures analysis are not exactly the same as the results obtained from a longitudinal analysis of covariance. This is caused by the adjustment for the

```
Mixed-effects ML regression                   Number of obs      =         416
Group variable: id                            Number of groups   =         150

                                              Obs per group:
                                                            min =           1
                                                            avg =         2.8
                                                            max =           3

                                              Wald chi2(6)       =       58.18
Log likelihood = -213.66378                   Prob > chi2        =      0.0000

------------------------------------------------------------------------------
   change_com |      Coef.   Std. Err.      z    P>|z|     [95% Conf. Interval]
--------------+---------------------------------------------------------------
 intervention |  -.1440671   .0789085    -1.83   0.068    -.2987249    .0105907
              |
         time |
            1 |   .0826913   .0527159     1.57   0.117    -.0206301    .1860126
            3 |   -.042738   .0525457    -0.81   0.416    -.1457256    .0602497
              |
        time# |
           c. |
 intervention |
            1 |    .040448   .0763355     0.53   0.596    -.1091668    .1900627
            3 |  -.0395289    .076004    -0.52   0.603     -.188494    .1094361
              |
     baseline |  -.4710729   .0778606    -6.05   0.000    -.6236767    -.318469
        _cons |   1.328167   .2740424     4.85   0.000     .7910532     1.86528
------------------------------------------------------------------------------


------------------------------------------------------------------------------
 Random-effects Parameters |   Estimate   Std. Err.     [95% Conf. Interval]
---------------------------+--------------------------------------------------
id: Identity               |
                var(_cons) |   .1138685   .0179887      .0835474    .1551939
---------------------------+--------------------------------------------------
              var(Residual)|   .0978093   .0085373      .0824295    .1160587
------------------------------------------------------------------------------
LR test vs. linear model: chibar2(01) = 100.99        Prob >= chibar2 = 0.0000
```

Output 3.20 Results of the longitudinal mixed model analysis of changes including an interaction between intervention and time with the second follow-up measurement as reference time point, adjusted for the baseline value

dependency of the repeated observations within the subject by adding a random intercept to the model. In the repeated measures analysis using all measurements as outcome, this random intercept variance is mostly a bit higher than in the longitudinal analysis of covariance. In the latter, part of the random intercept variance is explained by the baseline value of the outcome which is included in the model. However, in the present example, this is not the case. Another difference between the alternative repeated measures analysis and the longitudinal analysis of covariance is that the standard errors of the effect estimates are a bit lower in the alternative repeated measures analysis. This has to do with the fact that the alternative repeated measures analysis includes more observations in the analysis. In the alternative repeated measures analysis, all four measurements are used as outcome, while in the longitudinal analysis of covariance, only the three follow-up measurements are used as outcome. The lower standard error in the alternative repeated measures

```
Mixed-effects ML regression                   Number of obs      =        416
Group variable: id                            Number of groups   =        150

                                              Obs per group:
                                                           min =          1
                                                           avg =        2.8
                                                           max =          3

                                              Wald chi2(6)       =      58.18
Log likelihood = -213.66378                   Prob > chi2        =     0.0000

--------------------------------------------------------------------------------
   change_com |    Coef.   Std. Err.      z    P>|z|    [95% Conf. Interval]
--------------+-----------------------------------------------------------------
 intervention | -.1835961   .0783288   -2.34   0.019    -.3371176   -.0300745
              |
         time |
            1 |  .1254292   .0530484    2.36   0.018     .0214562    .2294022
            2 |   .042738   .0525457    0.81   0.416    -.0602497    .1457256
              |
        time# |
           c. |
 intervention |
            1 |  .0799769   .0760742    1.05   0.293    -.0691258    .2290796
            2 |  .0395289    .076004    0.52   0.603    -.1094361     .188494
              |
     baseline | -.4710729   .0778606   -6.05   0.000    -.6236767    -.318469
        _cons |  1.285429   .2749108    4.68   0.000     .7466132    1.824244
--------------------------------------------------------------------------------


--------------------------------------------------------------------------------
 Random-effects Parameters  |   Estimate   Std. Err.    [95% Conf. Interval]
----------------------------+---------------------------------------------------
id: Identity                |
                 var(_cons) |   .1138685   .0179887     .0835474    .1551939
----------------------------+---------------------------------------------------
               var(Residual)|   .0978093   .0085373     .0824295    .1160587
--------------------------------------------------------------------------------
LR test vs. linear model: chibar2(01) = 100.99        Prob >= chibar2 = 0.0000
```

Output 3.21 Results of the longitudinal mixed model analysis of changes including an interaction between intervention and time with the third follow-up measurement as reference time point, adjusted for the baseline value

Table 3.7 Overview of overall effect estimates on average over time, 95% confidence intervals (CI), and p-values obtained from the different analyses

	Effect	95% CI	p-value
Longitudinal analysis of covariance	−0.14	−0.27 to −0.01	0.03
Repeated measures	−0.25	−0.37 to −0.12	<0.001
Alternative repeated measures	−0.15	−0.25 to −0.05	0.004
Analysis of changes			
Without adjustment for baseline	−0.05	−0.19 to 0.09	0.47
With adjustment for baseline	−0.14	−0.27 to −0.01	0.03

Table 3.8 Overview of effect estimates at the different follow-up measurements, 95% confidence intervals (CI), and p-values obtained from the different analyses

	Effect	95% CI	p-value
Longitudinal analysis of covariance			
First follow-up	−0.10	−0.26 to 0.05	0.19
Second follow-up	−0.14	−0.30 to 0.01	0.07
Third follow-up	−0.18	−0.34 to −0.03	0.02
Repeated measures			
First follow-up	−0.22	−0.38 to −0.06	0.006
Second follow-up	−0.27	−0.43 to −0.11	0.001
Third follow-up	−0.30	−0.46 to −0.14	<0.001
Alternative repeated measures			
First follow-up	−0.11	−0.24 to 0.03	0.12
Second follow-up	−0.16	−0.30 to −0.02	0.03
Third follow-up	−0.19	−0.32 to −0.05	0.008
Analysis of changes			
Without adjustment for baseline			
First follow-up	−0.01	−0.18 to 0.15	0.87
Second follow-up	−0.06	−0.22 to 0.11	0.51
Third follow-up	−0.10	−0.26 to 0.07	0.24
With adjustment for baseline			
First follow-up	−0.10	−0.26 to 0.05	0.19
Second follow-up	−0.14	−0.30 to 0.01	0.07
Third follow-up	−0.18	−0.34 to −0.03	0.02

analysis is, however, maybe invalid, because the observations at baseline are not related to the intervention. And although the inclusion of too many observations is counteracted by the correlation between the repeated measurements (Twisk, 2013, 2018), it still leads to a slight underestimation of the standard error.

3.6   Recommendation

To estimate an intervention effect in an RCT with more than one follow-up measurement, the analysis has to be adjusted for the baseline value of the outcome variable. A proper adjustment is not achieved by performing a standard repeated measures analysis with the baseline value as part of the outcome variable or by the analysis of changes without adjusting for the baseline value. It is advised to use either a longitudinal analysis of covariance (or its mathematical equivalent, analysis of changes with an adjustment for the baseline value) or an alternative repeated measures analysis.

3.7   Should the Analysis Be Adjusted for Time?

In the literature there is some discussion whether the analysis to obtain the overall effect of the intervention on average over time should be adjusted for the time variable. Some researchers believe that the time variable should always be part of the model. The main argument for this is that there is always a development over time in the outcome variable. So, time is related to the outcome, and, therefore, the analysis should be adjusted for the time variable. Although the first part of this argument is true, mostly there is a development over time in the outcome variable, and it should be realized that adding a variable to a regression model can have an influence on the regression coefficient of interest only when the variable is related to both the outcome and the independent variable. In this case, the time variable is related to the outcome, but not to the independent variable. In a regular RCT, the intervention and control groups are measured at the same time points, so there is no relationship between the intervention variable and time. Therefore, the adjustment for the time variable in the analysis to obtain the overall effect of the intervention on average over time does not make sense.

3.8   Alternative Repeated Measures for the Analysis of an RCT with One Follow-Up Measurement

The alternative repeated measures analysis (i.e., the mixed model analysis with both the baseline and the follow-up measurements as outcome and without the intervention variable as independent variable) can also be used in the example with only one follow-up measurement (see Table 2.2). Output 3.22 shows the results of this analysis performed on the example with only one follow-up measurement for total serum cholesterol (Output 3.22a) and the physical activity index (Output 3.22b).

The two effect estimates can be directly derived from the outputs of the alternative repeated measures analyses. For total serum cholesterol, the effect estimate equals -0.141 with a 95% confidence interval ranging from -0.296 to 0.014 and with a corresponding p-value $= 0.07$. For the physical activity index, the effect estimate equals 0.308 with a 95% confidence interval ranging from 0.130 to 0.486 and a corresponding p-value <0.001. In Chap. 2, the effect estimates of this example were based on an analysis of covariance, and they were respectively -0.137 and

```
Mixed-effects ML regression                    Number of obs      =       521
Group variable: id                             Number of groups   =       299

                                               Obs per group:
                                                            min =         1
                                                            avg =       1.7
                                                            max =         2

                                               Wald chi2(2)       =      7.83
Log likelihood = -615.61809                    Prob > chi2        =    0.0200

-----------------------------------------------------------------------------
        chol |      Coef.   Std. Err.      z    P>|z|     [95% Conf. Interval]
-------------+---------------------------------------------------------------
interven_time| -.1411914   .0790782    -1.79   0.074    -.2961817     .013799
        time | -.0217071   .0555536    -0.39   0.696    -.1305903     .087176
       _cons |  5.460468   .0567095    96.29   0.000      5.34932    5.571617
-----------------------------------------------------------------------------


-----------------------------------------------------------------------------
  Random-effects Parameters  |   Estimate   Std. Err.     [95% Conf. Interval]
-----------------------------+-----------------------------------------------
id: Identity                 |
                var(_cons)   |   .7693342   .0738162      .6374467    .9285092
-----------------------------+-----------------------------------------------
              var(Residual)  |   .1922402   .0183182      .1594905    .2317146
-----------------------------------------------------------------------------
LR test vs. linear model: chibar2(01) = 218.98        Prob >= chibar2 = 0.0000
```

Output 3.22a Results of the alternative repeated measures mixed model analysis for total serum cholesterol in the example with only one follow-up measurement

```
Mixed-effects ML regression                    Number of obs      =       514
Group variable: id                             Number of groups   =       297

                                               Obs per group:
                                                            min =         1
                                                            avg =       1.7
                                                            max =         2

                                               Wald chi2(2)       =     11.51
Log likelihood = -655.82605                    Prob > chi2        =    0.0032

-----------------------------------------------------------------------------
         act |      Coef.   Std. Err.      z    P>|z|     [95% Conf. Interval]
-------------+---------------------------------------------------------------
interven_time|  .3077802   .0908019     3.39   0.001     .1298117    .4857486
        time | -.1350004   .0632529    -2.13   0.033    -.2589738    -.011027
       _cons |  5.587473   .0609397    91.69   0.000     5.468033    5.706912
-----------------------------------------------------------------------------


-----------------------------------------------------------------------------
  Random-effects Parameters  |   Estimate   Std. Err.     [95% Conf. Interval]
-----------------------------+-----------------------------------------------
id: Identity                 |
                var(_cons)   |    .837105   .082907       .6894088   1.016443
-----------------------------+-----------------------------------------------
              var(Residual)  |    .254875   .0244064      .2112602    .3074942
-----------------------------------------------------------------------------
LR test vs. linear model: chibar2(01) = 192.35        Prob >= chibar2 = 0.0000
```

Output 3.22b Results of the alternative repeated measures mixed model analysis for the physical activity index in the example with only one follow-up measurement

0.347. The (small) differences are due to the fact that in the alternative repeated measures analysis, subjects with only a baseline value are included in the analysis, while in the analysis of covariance, they are not. Therefore, the number of observations analyzed with the two methods is different. From Output 3.22 it can be seen that the number of subjects included in the two alternative repeated measures analyses were respectively 299 and 297, while in Chap. 2 (Outputs 2.1 and 2.2) it could be seen that the number of subjects analyzed in the longitudinal analysis of covariance was equal to 222 and 217, respectively.

Chapter 4
Analysis of Data from a Cluster RCT

4.1 Introduction

The most efficient way to perform the randomization within an RCT is on the subject level. Each subject is randomized into either the intervention group or the control group. However, in some situations it is not possible to randomize the individual subjects, but the randomization has to be performed on a higher level. For instance, the randomization can be performed on the hospital level (i.e., intervention hospitals versus control hospitals), nursery home level, or medical doctor level. Also in a nonmedical setting, it is possible to perform randomization on a higher level than the subject. When an intervention is applied on school children, the randomization can be performed on school level. Another example is when an intervention is applied to whole families, the randomization should be performed on family level. The reason for performing a cluster randomization is mostly a logistic one but sometimes also to prevent contamination. When the randomization is performed on a higher level, the RCT becomes a cluster RCT (see Fig. 4.1).

When the data of a cluster RCT is analyzed, the statistical methods are slightly more complicated than the methods used for analyzing the data from an RCT with individual randomization. The problem with the analysis of data from a cluster RCT is the fact that the observations of subjects belonging to the same cluster (e.g., hospital, nursery home, medical doctor, school, or family) are not independent of each other. Independency of observations is one of the key assumptions in regular statistical analysis. So, when data of a cluster RCT is analyzed, the dependency of the observations within the cluster must be taken into account. The most simple way of dealing with that dependency is to adjust for the cluster variable, i.e., adjust for the hospital, the nursery home, medical doctor, school, or family. That adjustment works well when the number of clusters is relatively low in comparison to the total number of subjects. When the number of clusters becomes large, the standard adjustment for the cluster variable is not possible anymore. It should be realized that in regular regression analysis, the adjustment for a cluster variable is performed by adding

J. W. R. Twisk, *Analysis of Data from Randomized Controlled Trials*,
https://doi.org/10.1007/978-3-030-81865-4_4

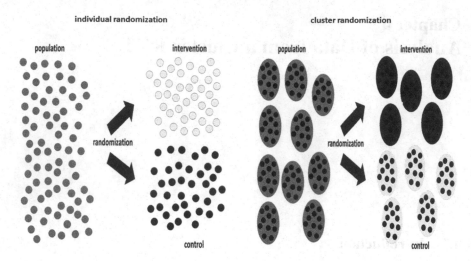

Fig. 4.1 Individual randomization versus cluster randomization

dummy variables to the regression model. Because the number of dummy variables equals the number of clusters minus 1, it is obvious that the more clusters there are, the less efficient the estimates of the regression model will be. More or less the same situation has already been discussed in Chap. 3 when the analysis of an RCT with more than one follow-up measurement was discussed. In that situation, there were dependent observations of the different follow-up measurements within a subject. Therefore, mixed model analyses were used as a very efficient way to deal with this dependency. The same holds for a cluster RCT. The general idea behind a mixed model analysis in a cluster RCT is that the adjustment for the cluster variable is performed by estimating only one parameter irrespective of the number of clusters. To understand the basic principles of a mixed model analysis in a cluster RCT, assume an RCT with only one follow-up measurement using analysis of covariance to estimate the intervention effect. That regression model includes an intercept, the intervention variable, and the baseline variable of the outcome. Suppose this model has to be adjusted for sex. This adjustment is performed by adding the variable sex to the model, but it actually means that for males and females, two different intercepts are estimated. The adjustment for the cluster variable in a cluster RCT is basically the same, i.e., for each cluster a separate intercept is estimated. Again, when the number of clusters is large in comparison to the number of subjects, the regular adjustment with the dummy variables is not efficient and therefore not possible. How is this adjustment performed in a mixed model analysis? Well, basically the efficient adjustment for the clusters is the same as the efficient adjustment for the subjects as has been described in Chap. 3 and contains three steps: (1) for each cluster a separate intercept is estimated (as in a regular adjustment), (2) a normal distribution is drawn over all the intercepts, and (3) from that normal distribution, the variance is estimated, and that variance is added to the regression model to adjust for the clustering. This variance is known as the random intercept variance on the cluster level. See for further details Twisk et al. (2018).

4.2 Example with One Follow-Up Measurement

The first example is a cluster RCT performed among 20 general practitioners (GPs) in order to evaluate the effectiveness of a new intervention to reduce pain. Pain was measured on a scale from 0 to 10, and unfortunately no baseline measurement was performed, so the analysis can only be performed on pain at the follow-up measurement without an adjustment for the baseline differences in pain between the groups. The randomization was done on GP level, meaning that the patients from 10 GPs were allocated to the new intervention, while the patients of the other 10 GPs were allocated to the control condition (i.e., usual care). Table 4.1 shows descriptive information for the example cluster RCT.

To illustrate the influence of the clustering on the results of the analysis, first an analysis is performed in which the dependency of the observations within the GP is ignored. Output 4.1 shows the results of the linear regression analysis.

It should be noted that the linear regression analysis is performed within a mixed model framework, without the adjustment for GP. This is basically the same as a regular linear regression analysis with pain at follow-up as outcome and the group variable as independent variable. The analysis without taking into account the dependency of the observations within the cluster is also known as a naive analysis. From Output 4.1 it can be seen that the intervention effect is -0.2424444. This effect

Table 4.1 Descriptive information (mean and standard deviation) regarding the cluster RCT with only one follow-up measurement

	N	Pain at the follow-up measurement
Intervention group	90	6.51 (0.86)
Control group	90	6.75 (0.89)

```
Mixed-effects ML regression                    Number of obs    =       180

                                               Wald chi2(1)     =      3.52
Log likelihood = -229.79376                    Prob > chi2      =    0.0608

-----------------------------------------------------------------------------
        pain |    Coef.   Std. Err.     z    P>|z|    [95% Conf. Interval]
-------------+---------------------------------------------------------------
intervention | -.2424444   .1292977   -1.88  0.061   -.4958633    .0109744
       _cons |  6.749778   .0914273   73.83  0.000    6.570584    6.928972
-----------------------------------------------------------------------------


-----------------------------------------------------------------------------
Random-effects Parameters  |  Estimate   Std. Err.    [95% Conf. Interval]
---------------------------+-------------------------------------------------
             var(Residual) |  .7523053   .0792999     .6118847    .9249508
-----------------------------------------------------------------------------
```

Output 4.1 Results of the linear regression analysis ignoring the dependency of the observations

```
Mixed-effects ML regression                 Number of obs    =        180
Group variable: gp                          Number of groups =         20

                                            Obs per group:
                                                         min =          8
                                                         avg =        9.0
                                                         max =         10

                                            Wald chi2(1)     =       1.43
Log likelihood = -220.09704                 Prob > chi2      =     0.2314

------------------------------------------------------------------------------
        pain |     Coef.   Std. Err.      z    P>|z|     [95% Conf. Interval]
-------------+----------------------------------------------------------------
intervention |  -.2574604   .2151456   -1.20   0.231    -.679138    .1642171
       _cons |   6.783696   .1521309   44.59   0.000    6.485525    7.081867
------------------------------------------------------------------------------


------------------------------------------------------------------------------
  Random-effects Parameters  |   Estimate   Std. Err.    [95% Conf. Interval]
-----------------------------+------------------------------------------------
gp: Identity                 |
                  var(_cons) |   .1656118    .073509    .0693863    .3952834
-----------------------------+------------------------------------------------
               var(Residual) |   .5871894   .0656448    .4716482    .7310352
------------------------------------------------------------------------------
LR test vs. linear model: chibar2(01) = 19.39         Prob >= chibar2 = 0.0000
```

Output 4.2 Results of the mixed model analysis taking into account the dependency of the observations within the GP

estimate is (of course) exactly the same as the difference between the two average pain values at the follow-up measurement between the two groups (see Table 4.1).

Second, a mixed model analysis is performed in which the dependency of the observations is taken into account by adding a random intercept on GP level to the model. Output 4.2 shows the result of this mixed model analysis.

In Chap. 3, it was already mentioned that the output of a mixed model analysis contains three parts. In the first part, some general information of the model is provided. It can be seen that there are 180 observations in 20 GPs and that on average there are 9 patients for each GP. Note that in this example the group variable is GP, while in Chap. 3 the group variable was id (the subject). In Chap. 3, follow-up measurements were clustered within the subject, while in this example, patients are clustered within the GP. In the first part of the output, also the log likelihood is given. The log likelihood is used for the likelihood ratio test, which can be used to compare models with each other.

The second part of Output 4.2 shows the fixed part of the model. It can be seen that the effect estimate (−0.2574604) is slightly different from the effect estimate obtained from the naive analysis. A more interesting finding is the fact that the standard error of the estimate is much higher in the mixed model analysis with a random intercept on GP level compared to the naive analysis (0.1292977 versus 0.2151456). The fact that the standard error is higher in a mixed model analysis with a random intercept on GP level is a general finding and has to do with the fact that part of the data is correlated. In a naive analysis, each individual patient provides 100% new information. In a mixed model analysis, on the other hand, the first patient of a GP provides 100% new information, but the second patient of that GP provides less information. Part of the information provided by the second patient was already provided by the first patient. The same holds for the third patient of the same GP, etc. Therefore, the total amount of information used in a mixed model analysis is less than the total amount of information used in a naive analysis. This leads to higher standard errors in the mixed model analysis with a random intercept on GP level. How much bigger the standard error will be depends on the magnitude of the correlation of the patient observations within the GP. This correlation is known as the intraclass correlation coefficient (ICC) and can be estimated by dividing the between group variance by the total variance. The variances are provided in the third part of the output of the mixed model analysis, the random part of the model. From Output 4.2 it can be seen that the between group variance equals 0.1656118. The total variance can be calculated by adding the between group variance to the residual variance $(0.1656118 + 0.5871894 = 0.7528012)$. Dividing the between group variance by the total variance $(0.1656118/0.7528012 = 0.22)$ gives an ICC of 22%.

It should be realized that in some situations the ICC can be very low and it is not necessary to take the correlation of the observations within the cluster into account. The necessity of taking the correlation into account can be evaluated by the likelihood ratio test. With the likelihood ratio test, two models are compared with each other. The test contains the difference between the -2 log likelihoods of the two models. This difference follows a chi-square distribution and the number of degrees of freedom of this chi-square distribution is equal to the difference in the number of parameters estimated by the two models. In the present example, the -2 log likelihood of the naive model equals -2 x $- 229.79376 = 459.58752$, while the -2 log likelihood of the mixed model analysis with a random intercept on GP level equals -2 x $- 220.09704 = 440.19408$. The difference between the two -2 log likelihoods equals 19.4. In a chi-square distribution with one degree of freedom (only the random intercept variance is additionally estimated in the mixed model analysis with a random intercept on GP level compared to the naive analysis), this 19.4 gives a highly significant p-value ($p < 0.001$). Note that the critical value of a chi-square distribution with one degree of freedom equals 3.84. So in this example it is necessary to take the correlation, (i.e., the clustering of the observations within the GP) into account. In the last line of Output 4.2, the result of this likelihood ratio test is also given. This is a typical feature of STATA. In the last line of the output of a mixed model analysis, the result of the likelihood ratio test comparing the particular model with the naive model (i.e., the model without any random coefficients) is provided.

4.3   Example with More Than One Follow-Up Measurement

The second example regarding the analysis of data from a cluster RCT is a cluster RCT performed in schools in order to improve the performance of students. In this particular study, schools were randomized into 24 intervention schools and 24 control schools. The number of students in the 24 control schools was 387, and the

Table 4.2 Descriptive information (mean and standard deviation) regarding the school example

	Baseline	First follow-up	Second follow-up
Intervention	25.2 (5.8)	30.9 (6.7)	31.8 (6.0)
Control	25.5 (5.8)	28.1 (6.6)	29.9 (6.2)

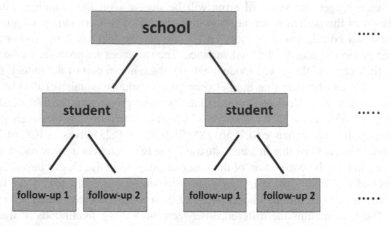

Fig. 4.2 Illustration of a three-level structure. The two follow-up measurements are clustered within the students, and the students are clustered within the schools

Table 4.3 Data structure needed to perform a longitudinal analysis of covariance in a cluster RCT

id	Outcome	Cluster	Time	Intervention	Baseline
1	Y_{t1}	1	1	1	Y_{t0}
1	Y_{t2}	1	2	1	Y_{t0}
1	Y_{t3}	1	3	1	Y_{t0}

number of students in the intervention schools was 500. In this cluster RCT, first a baseline measurement was performed. After one school year, the first follow-up measurement was performed, and after two school years, the second follow-up measurement was performed. The performance of the students was quantified with an overall test result, which score theoretically ranges between 0 and 50. Table 4.2 shows the descriptive information regarding this example.

In this example there are basically two different levels of correlated data. Firstly, the two follow-up measurements within the same student are correlated (see Chap. 3), and, secondly, there are correlated observations of the students within the school. Therefore, the data has a three-level structure; follow-up measurements are clustered within the students and the students are clustered within the schools (see Fig. 4.2).

In this example, there was a baseline measurement, so the analyses were adjusted for the baseline value of the outcome, i.e., a longitudinal analysis of covariance was used (see Chap. 3). Table 4.3 shows the structure of the data used to estimate the parameters for the longitudinal analysis of covariance in a cluster RCT.

```
Mixed-effects ML regression                    Number of obs      =        1,747
Group variable: student                        Number of groups   =          887

                                               Obs per group:
                                                            min =            1
                                                            avg =          2.0
                                                            max =            2

                                               Wald chi2(2)       =       388.16
Log likelihood = -4829.0365                    Prob > chi2        =       0.0000

---------------------------------------------------------------------------------
 performance |     Coef.   Std. Err.      z    P>|z|     [95% Conf. Interval]
-------------+-------------------------------------------------------------------
    baseline |   .5690345   .0308448    18.45   0.000     .5085797    .6294893
       group |   2.631033   .3597586     7.31   0.000     1.925919    3.336147
       _cons |   14.36098   .8317136    17.27   0.000     12.73086    15.99111
---------------------------------------------------------------------------------


---------------------------------------------------------------------------------
  Random-effects Parameters  |   Estimate   Std. Err.    [95% Conf. Interval]
-----------------------------+---------------------------------------------------
student: Identity            |
               var(_cons)    |   26.26482   1.342667     23.76079    29.03275
-----------------------------+---------------------------------------------------
              var(Residual)  |   3.773119   .181966      3.432809    4.147165
---------------------------------------------------------------------------------
LR test vs. linear model: chibar2(01) = 1242.16        Prob >= chibar2 = 0.0000
```

Output 4.3   Results of the longitudinal mixed model analysis of covariance

The first step in the analysis is a longitudinal mixed model analysis of covariance to obtain an overall intervention effect on average over time. In this first analysis, no adjustment is made for the clustering on school level. Output 4.3 shows the result of this analysis.

From the first part of Output 4.3, it can be seen that there are 1747 observations on 887 students, so for almost all students, there are two follow-up measurements. In the second part of the output, the regression coefficient for the group variable provides the overall intervention effect on average over time. So, the intervention group has (on average over time) a performance score which is 2.631033 points higher than the control group. This difference is adjusted for the baseline value, so the estimated difference is not influenced by regression to the mean (see Chaps. 2 and 3). Besides the effect estimate, the output also provides the standard error of the effect estimate, the 95% confidence interval around the effect estimate (which can be calculated by the effect estimate ± 1.96 x standard error), and the corresponding p-value. The latter is based on the z-value which is calculated by dividing the effect estimate by its standard error.

The last part of the output shows the random part of the model. In this part the random intercept variance on the student level is given. From this variance the ICC for the two follow-up measurements within the student can be calculated. From the estimated model, the ICC is equal to $26.26482/(26.26482 + 3.773119) = 0.87$. This indicates that there is an average correlation of 87% between the two follow-up measurements within the student. Although this correlation seems to be very high, it is often observed in longitudinal studies.

```
Mixed-effects ML regression                    Number of obs      =      1,747

------------------------------------------------------------
            |    No. of         Observations per Group
Group Variable |    Groups    Minimum    Average    Maximum
---------------+--------------------------------------------
      school |      48          10        36.4        124
     student |     887           1         2.0          2
------------------------------------------------------------

                                               Wald chi2(2)       =     358.73
Log likelihood = -4796.2925                    Prob > chi2        =     0.0000

------------------------------------------------------------------------------
performance |    Coef.    Std. Err.      z     P>|z|    [95% Conf. Interval]
------------+-----------------------------------------------------------------
   baseline |  .5684545   .0304715     18.66   0.000    .5087314     .6281775
      group |  2.346147   .6661906      3.52   0.000    1.040438     3.651857
      _cons |  14.6978    .9126499     16.10   0.000    12.90904     16.48656
------------------------------------------------------------------------------


------------------------------------------------------------------------------
Random-effects Parameters  |   Estimate   Std. Err.    [95% Conf. Interval]
---------------------------+--------------------------------------------------
school: Identity           |
               var(_cons)  |   3.73768    1.077773     2.124004     6.57732
---------------------------+--------------------------------------------------
student: Identity          |
               var(_cons)  |   22.53644   1.196804     20.3087      25.00856
---------------------------+--------------------------------------------------
           var(Residual)  |   3.769866   .1816596     3.430117     4.143268
------------------------------------------------------------------------------
LR test vs. linear model: chi2(2) = 1307.65          Prob > chi2 = 0.0000
```

Output 4.4 Results of the longitudinal mixed model analysis of covariance taking into account the dependency of the observations within schools

In the next step of the analysis, also an adjustment is made for the correlated observations within the schools. Output 4.4 shows the result of this analysis with both a random intercept on student level and a random intercept on school level.

In Output 4.4 it can be seen that a model with a three-level structure is analyzed. It can be seen that there are 48 schools involved in the study and that on average there are 36.4 students in each school. The second part of the output shows the fixed part of the model, and the regression coefficient for the group variable indicates (again) the overall effect estimate on average over time. The effect estimate (2.346147) is slightly different from the one obtained from the analysis without an adjustment for the correlated observations within the school. More striking is the difference in the estimated standard error of the effect estimates, 0.3597586 obtained from the analysis without the adjustment for the correlated observations within the schools and 0.6661906 obtained from the analysis with the adjustment for the correlated observations within the schools. In Sect. 4.2 it was already explained why the standard errors become bigger when an adjustment is made for the correlated observations within a cluster variable. The total amount of information used in the analysis is less when the correlations are taken into account and less information leads to higher standard errors. Also in this three-level model, the necessity of adjusting for (in this example) the school can be evaluated by the likelihood ratio test (see Sect. 4.2). In this case the -2 log likelihood of the model with only an adjustment for the correlated follow-up measurements within the student must be compared with the -2 log likelihood of the model with both an adjustment for the correlated follow-up measurements and the correlated observations of the students within the schools. The -2 log likelihood of the first model equals -2 x $- 4829.0365 = 9658.073$, while the -2 log likelihood of the second model equals -2 x $- 4796.2925 = 9592.585$. The difference between the two -2 log likelihoods is 65.488. This difference must be evaluated on a chi-square distribution with one degree of freedom and is therefore highly significant (note again that the critical value of a chi-square distribution with one degree of freedom is 3.84). Because of this highly significant p-value, it can be concluded that the effect estimate must be derived from the model with both a random intercept on the student level and a random intercept on the school level.

In Chap. 3, it was already discussed that in an RCT with more than one follow-up measurement, the next step in the analysis is to estimate the effects of the intervention at the different follow-up measurements. Therefore, time and the interaction between the group variable and time must be added to the longitudinal analysis of covariance. Because the model with a random intercept on student level and a random intercept on school level was the best way to estimate the effect of the intervention, the effects of the intervention at the two follow-up measurements were also estimated with this three-level model. Output 4.5 shows the results of the analysis with the first follow-up measurement as reference time point, and Output 4.6 shows the result of the analysis with the second follow-up measurement as reference time point.

It was already discussed in Chap. 3, that the effect estimate for the first follow-up measurement is provided by the regression coefficient for the group variable from the analysis with the first follow-up measurement as reference time point (Output 4.5). This regression coefficient equals 2.674009, with a 95% confidence interval ranging from 1.379141 to 3.968877 and a corresponding p-value <0.001. The effect estimate for the second follow-up measurement is slightly lower and is provided by the regression coefficient for the group variable from the analysis with the second follow-up measurement as reference time point (Output 4.6). This regression coefficient equals 1.956215, with a 95% confidence interval ranging from 0.6601865 to 3.252243 and a corresponding p-value of 0.003.

4.4 Comment

In the examples of this chapter, the likelihood ratio rest was used to evaluate the necessity of adding a random intercept on the cluster level to the model. It should be noted that in the examples the likelihood ratio test was not used to evaluate the necessity of adding a random intercept on the student level. This was done on

```
Mixed-effects ML regression                    Number of obs     =        1,747
-----------------------------------------------------------------
               |  No. of       Observations per Group
 Group Variable |  Groups    Minimum    Average    Maximum
----------------+------------------------------------------------
        school |     48        10        36.4        124
       student |    887         1         2.0          2
-----------------------------------------------------------------
                                               Wald chi2(4)      =       578.75
Log likelihood = -4698.4977                    Prob > chi2       =       0.0000

-----------------------------------------------------------------------------
 performance |    Coef.    Std. Err.      z     P>|z|     [95% Conf. Interval]
-------------+---------------------------------------------------------------
    baseline |  .5688543   .0304574    18.68   0.000      .509159     .6285497
       group |  2.674009   .6606592     4.05   0.000     1.379141    3.968877
      2.time |  1.603794   .1291838    12.41   0.000     1.350599     1.85699
             |
time#c.group |
           2 | -.7177943   .1694578    -4.24   0.000    -1.049925   -.3856631
             |
       _cons |  13.91834   .9105831    15.29   0.000     12.13363    15.70305
-----------------------------------------------------------------------------


-----------------------------------------------------------------------------
 Random-effects Parameters  |   Estimate   Std. Err.    [95% Conf. Interval]
----------------------------+------------------------------------------------
school: Identity            |
                var(_cons)  |   3.570421   1.045435     2.011333    6.33804
----------------------------+------------------------------------------------
student: Identity           |
                var(_cons)  |   22.94109   1.196509     20.71186    25.41026
----------------------------+------------------------------------------------
             var(Residual)  |   3.00687    .1449154     2.735843    3.304746
-----------------------------------------------------------------------------
LR test vs. linear model: chi2(2) = 1475.51          Prob > chi2 = 0.0000
```

Output 4.5 Results of the longitudinal mixed model analysis of covariance including an interaction between the group variable and time with the first follow-up as reference time point

purpose because a longitudinal data analysis which ignores the dependency of the follow-up measurements within the subject is theoretically wrong. So, when there is more than one follow-up measurement analyzed in one model, a random intercept on subject level is always added to the model.

```
Mixed-effects ML regression                    Number of obs     =      1,747

-----------------------------------------------------------------
             |   No. of        Observations per Group
Group Variable |   Groups    Minimum    Average   Maximum
---------------+-------------------------------------------------
      school |       48         10       36.4       124
     student |      887          1        2.0         2
-----------------------------------------------------------------

                                               Wald chi2(4)     =     578.75
Log likelihood = -4698.4977                    Prob > chi2      =     0.0000

--------------------------------------------------------------------------------
performance |     Coef.   Std. Err.      z    P>|z|     [95% Conf. Interval]
------------+-------------------------------------------------------------------
   baseline |   .5688543   .0304574    18.68   0.000     .509159    .6285497
      group |   1.956215   .6612511     2.96   0.003    .6601865    3.252243
     1.time |  -1.603794   .1291838   -12.41   0.000    -1.85699   -1.350599
            |
time#c.group |
          1 |   .7177943   .1694578     4.24   0.000    .3856631    1.049925
            |
      _cons |   15.52214   .9108684    17.04   0.000    13.73687    17.30741
--------------------------------------------------------------------------------


--------------------------------------------------------------------------------
Random-effects Parameters |  Estimate   Std. Err.    [95% Conf. Interval]
--------------------------+-----------------------------------------------------
school: Identity          |
              var(_cons) |  3.570421   1.045435    2.011333     6.33804
--------------------------+-----------------------------------------------------
student: Identity         |
              var(_cons) |  22.94109   1.196509    20.71186    25.41026
--------------------------+-----------------------------------------------------
            var(Residual) |   3.00687    .1449154   2.735843    3.304746
--------------------------------------------------------------------------------
LR test vs. linear model: chi2(2) = 1475.51              Prob > chi2 = 0.0000
```

Output 4.6 Results of the longitudinal mixed model analysis of covariance including an interaction between the group variable and time with the second follow-up as reference time point

Chapter 5
Analysis of Data from a Cross-Over Trial

5.1 Introduction

A cross-over trial is characterized by the situation that the subject receives both the intervention and the control condition (see Fig. 5.1). Basically this means that the subject acts as its own control. The randomization in a cross-over trial is related to the sequence in which the intervention and control condition are delivered.

Because of the fact that in a cross-over trial the subject receives both conditions, the analysis is slightly more complicated than the analysis of a regular RCT. Table 5.1 shows the data structure needed to analyze the data from a cross-over trial.

An important issue in cross-over trials is the wash-out period. The wash-out period is the period between the ending of the first phase of the sequence and the start of the second phase. It is obvious that the wash-out period must be long enough to let the subjects return to their baseline situation. Because of this, cross-over trials are especially suitable for analyzing interventions that has a short-term effect only. Another important issue in cross-over trials is the possibility for a carry-over effect. A carry-over effect indicates that the effect of the intervention in the intervention phase is carried over to the next phase in which the subject will receive the control condition. It is obvious that the possibility of a carry-over effect should be part of the analysis, because the existence of a carry-over effect can highly bias the final effect estimate of the intervention.

Because each subject receives both the intervention and the control condition, the estimated intervention effect has a different interpretation than in a regular RCT. Due to the fact that each subject acts as its own control, the interpretation of the intervention effect is within subjects, while the interpretation of the intervention effect in a regular RCT is between subjects (Twisk, 2013, 2018).

In Chap. 3, it was mentioned that with a linear mixed model analysis, an adjustment is made for the dependency of the observations within the subject. In a cross-over this is basically the same; a random intercept on the subject level has to be added to the model to adjust for this dependency. However, it is also possible that the

J. W. R. Twisk, *Analysis of Data from Randomized Controlled Trials*,
https://doi.org/10.1007/978-3-030-81865-4_5

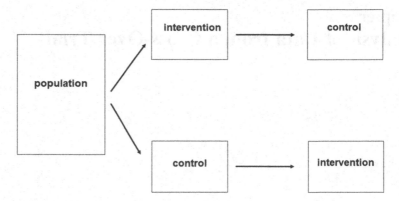

Fig. 5.1 Design of a cross-over trial

Table 5.1 Data structure
needed to perform an analysis
of data from a cross-over trial

id	Outcome	Time	Intervention	Baseline	Sequence[a]
1	Y_{t1}	0	1	Y_{r01}	1
1	Y_{t2}	1	0	Y_{r02}	1
2	Y_{t1}	0	0	Y_{r01}	0
2	Y_{t2}	1	1	Y_{r02}	0

[a]Sequence 1 indicates that a subject started with the intervention
condition followed by the control condition

effect of the intervention is different for the different subjects. In a cross-over trial, it
is possible to include this difference in intervention effect between subjects to the
model. Basically, there is a sort of interaction between the intervention variable and
the subject. In Chap. 3, it was discussed that a random intercept has to be added to
the model to adjust for the dependency of the (follow-up) observations within the
subject. Adding a random intercept to the model was a very efficient way to adjust
for the correlated observations within the subject. This efficient method was needed
because an adjustment for the subject by, for instance, adding a dummy variable for
each subject is not possible. Basically, the same holds for the interaction between the
intervention and the subject. It is also not possible to add an interaction term between
the intervention variable and the dummy variable for each subject to the model.
Comparable to the three-step approach to adjust for the subject described in Chap. 3,
also regarding the interaction between the intervention and the subject a three-step
approach is used. First, for each subject a regression coefficient for the intervention
is estimated. Second, a normal distribution is drawn over all the regression coefficients, and, third, the variance of this normal distribution is calculated. This variance
is known as the random slope variance. In Sect. 3.4, the random slope was already
introduced. In that section it was mentioned that a random slope for the intervention
was only possible in a situation where the intervention variable is time-dependent. In
a cross-over trial this is the case, so, therefore, in a cross-over trial, a random slope
for the intervention variable can be added to the model.

5.2 Example

The example contains a cross-over trial to evaluate the effectiveness of a new treatment to reduce pain in 54 patients with chronic pain. The sequence of receiving the treatment or control condition was randomized. Table 5.2 shows the descriptive information of the example dataset.

From the descriptive information provided in Table 5.2, it can be seen that the decrease in pain is stronger after the treatment condition than after the control condition. Output 5.1 shows the result of the longitudinal mixed model analysis in which the treatment and control condition are compared to each other regarding pain after treatment or control.

Output 5.1 looks similar to the outputs shown in the foregoing chapters. Again, the output contains three parts. The first part shows some overall model information including the log likelihood, the number of subjects, and the number of measurements. From this part it can be seen that not all patients received both the treatment and control condition. This is not really a problem, because mixed model analysis is

Table 5.2 Descriptive information (mean and standard deviation) of the example cross-over trial

	Pain before	Pain after
Control condition	2.49 (0.76)	2.14 (0.69)
Treatment condition	2.43 (0.73)	1.80 (0.70)

```
Mixed-effects ML regression                  Number of obs      =        101
Group variable: patient                      Number of groups   =         54

                                             Obs per group:
                                                          min =          1
                                                          avg =        1.9
                                                          max =          2

                                             Wald chi2(1)       =      14.22
Log likelihood = -95.665568                  Prob > chi2        =     0.0002

------------------------------------------------------------------------------
        pain |     Coef.   Std. Err.      z    P>|z|    [95% Conf. Interval]
-------------+----------------------------------------------------------------
   treatment |  -.3391977   .0899588    -3.77   0.000   -.5155137   -.1628817
       _cons |   2.121772   .0954243    22.24   0.000    1.934743     2.3088
------------------------------------------------------------------------------


------------------------------------------------------------------------------
  Random-effects Parameters  |   Estimate   Std. Err.    [95% Conf. Interval]
-----------------------------+------------------------------------------------
patient: Identity            |
               var(_cons)    |   .2773686   .0766366     .161388     .476698
-----------------------------+------------------------------------------------
            var(Residual)    |   .1960275   .0401051    .1312714    .2927276
------------------------------------------------------------------------------
LR test vs. linear model: chibar2(01) = 20.24      Prob >= chibar2 = 0.0000
```

Output 5.1 Results of a longitudinal mixed model analysis to estimate the treatment effect in the example cross-over trial a method that can handle missing data in a very efficient way (Twisk, 2013; Twisk et al., 2013).

The second part of the output shows the fixed part of the model with the regression coefficients. The coefficient for treatment (-0.3391977) indicates the difference in pain between the treatment and the control condition. The output also gives the 95% confidence interval around the treatment effect (ranging from -0.5155137 to -0.1628817) and the corresponding p-value (<0.001). In the third part of the output, the random part of the model is shown. This part includes the random intercept variance (0.2773686) and the remaining residual variance (0.1960275).

As has been mentioned before, it should be realized that the analysis of data from a cross-over trial is slightly different from the analysis of a regular RCT, which was described in the foregoing chapters. Because in a cross-over trial the patient acts as its own control, the treatment variable is a time-dependent variable, which is not the case in a regular RCT. The fact that the treatment variable is time-dependent has a few implications. The first implication is the interpretation of the treatment effect. It has already been mentioned that the treatment effect interpretation is a within patient interpretation, i.e., it indicates the difference between the treatment and control condition within the patient. In a regular RCT, the interpretation of the treatment effect is a between patient interpretation, i.e., it indicates the difference between the treatment condition and the control condition on average between the patients. It should be realized that when some of the patients have a missing value for one of the two conditions, the estimated treatment effect does not have a 100% within patient interpretation anymore. However, assuming that the number of missing observations is not that high, this difference is ignorable.

The second implication is that it is possible to model a random slope for treatment, which means that possible different treatment effects for patients can be modeled (see Sect. 5.1). Output 5.2 shows the result of the analysis including a random slope for treatment.

The difference between Outputs 5.1 and 5.2 can be found in the random part of the model. In Output 5.1 the results of a model with only a random intercept were provided, while in Output 5.2 the results of a model with both a random intercept and a random slope for treatment are given. Besides the random slope variance (var (treatm~t)), also the covariance between the random intercept and the random slope for treatment is given (cov(treatm~t,_cons). This covariance indicates the relationship between the average value of pain for a particular patient and the treatment effect for that patient. It makes a lot of sense to model that covariance in combination with the random slope for treatment, because it is highly plausible that the effect of the treatment for a particular patient depends on the average pain value for that particular patient. When a random slope is added to the model, the likelihood ratio test can be used to evaluate whether or not this random slope was necessary. Therefore, the -2 log likelihood of the model with only a random intercept must be compared with the -2 log likelihood of the model with a random intercept, a random slope, and the covariance between the random intercept and the random slope. The difference between the two -2 log likelihoods follows then a chi-square

```
Mixed-effects ML regression                    Number of obs      =        101
Group variable: patient                        Number of groups   =         54

                                               Obs per group:
                                                            min =          1
                                                            avg =        1.9
                                                            max =          2

                                               Wald chi2(1)       =      14.23
Log likelihood = -95.664179                    Prob > chi2        =     0.0002

-------------------------------------------------------------------------------
       pain |      Coef.   Std. Err.      z    P>|z|     [95% Conf. Interval]
------------+------------------------------------------------------------------
  treatment |  -.3394054   .0899669    -3.77   0.000    -.5157374   -.1630735
      _cons |   2.121869   .0951368    22.30   0.000     1.935404    2.308334
-------------------------------------------------------------------------------


-------------------------------------------------------------------------------
  Random-effects Parameters  |   Estimate   Std. Err.    [95% Conf. Interval]
-----------------------------+-------------------------------------------------
patient: Unstructured        |
            var(treatm~t)    |    .265158   32.23002     9.1e-105     7.7e+102
            var(_cons)       |   .4070813   16.11539     8.18e-35     2.03e+33
       cov(treatm~t,_cons)   |  -.1297106    16.1152    -31.71491     31.45549
-----------------------------+-------------------------------------------------
            var(Residual)    |   .0634666   16.11501     4.7e-218     8.6e+214
-------------------------------------------------------------------------------
LR test vs. linear model: chi2(3) = 20.24           Prob > chi2 =      0.0002
```

Output 5.2 Results of a longitudinal mixed model analysis to estimate the treatment effect in the example cross-over trial including a random slope for treatment

distribution with two degrees of freedom (because besides the random slope variance, also the covariance between random intercept and random slope is estimated), and the critical value of this chi-square distribution with two degrees of freedom is 5.99. If the -2 log likelihoods of the two models are compared to each other, it can be seen that they are almost the same; the difference between the two is 0.003. This is far from significant, so in this particular situation, it is not necessary to add a random slope for treatment to the model.

Continuing with a model with only a random intercept, several additional analyses can be performed. It has been mentioned before that one of the key issues in a cross-over trial is a possible carry-over effect. To get some insight in a possible carry-over effect, the descriptive information shown in Table 5.2 is stratified for the two randomized sequences (see Table 5.3).

From Table 5.3 it can be seen that the average pain before the measurement for the treatment condition was much higher for the patients who started the cross-over trial with the control condition compared to the patients who started the cross-over trial with the treatment condition. This suggest a carry-over effect, because part of the intervention effect in the first phase seems to be carried over to the second phase in which these patients received the control condition. In general, to evaluate the influence of the sequence on the estimated intervention effect, sequence can be added to the model as a possible effect modifier. Analyzing sequence as a possible confounder makes no sense, because treatment and sequence are not related to each

Table 5.3 Descriptive information (mean and standard deviation) of the example cross-over trial stratified for sequence[a]

	Pain before	Pain after
Control condition		
Sequence = 0	2.48 (0.90)	2.13 (0.81)
Sequence = 1	2.5 (0.64)	2.14 (0.59)
Treatment condition		
Sequence = 0	2.31 (0.79)	1.8 (0.65)
Sequence = 1	2.56 (0.65)	1.8 (0.76)

[a]Sequence = 0 indicates that a patient started with the control condition followed by the treatment condition; sequence = 1 indicates that a patient started with the treatment condition followed by the control condition

```
Mixed-effects ML regression              Number of obs      =       101
Group variable: patient                  Number of groups   =        54

                                         Obs per group:
                                                      min =         1
                                                      avg =       1.9

                                         Wald chi2(2)       =     14.26
Log likelihood = -95.648795              Prob > chi2        =    0.0008

------------------------------------------------------------------------------
       pain |    Coef.    Std. Err.      z    P>|z|    [95% Conf. Interval]
------------+-----------------------------------------------------------------
  treatment | -.3385413   .0900034    -3.76   0.000   -.5149448   -.1621379
   sequence |  .0310145   .1693117     0.18   0.855   -.3008304    .3628593
      _cons |  2.105285   .1311482    16.05   0.000    1.848239    2.362331
------------------------------------------------------------------------------


------------------------------------------------------------------------------
  Random-effects Parameters  |   Estimate   Std. Err.    [95% Conf. Interval]
-----------------------------+------------------------------------------------
id: Identity                 |
                  var(_cons) |   .2773998   .0765876     .161472     .4765575
-----------------------------+------------------------------------------------
               var(Residual) |   .1959079   .0400661     .1312105    .2925065
------------------------------------------------------------------------------
LR test vs. linear model: chibar2(01) = 20.27       Prob >= chibar2 = 0.0000
```

Output 5.3 Results of a longitudinal mixed model analysis to estimate the treatment effect in the example cross-over trial with an adjustment for sequence

other, and, therefore, sequence cannot be a confounder. To illustrate this (i.e., to analyze the possible confounding effect of the sequence), sequence is added to the model as a covariate. Output 5.3 shows the results of this analysis.

Whether or not the adjustment for sequence is necessary can be evaluated by comparing the treatment effect estimate from the model without the adjustment with the treatment effect estimate from the model with the adjustment. As expected, the two estimated treatment effects are almost the same (-0.3391977 versus -0.3385413). The fact that the two effects estimated are not exactly the same is caused by the fact that not all patients received both conditions.

```
Mixed-effects ML regression                        Number of obs     =         101
Group variable: patient                            Number of groups  =          54

                                                   Obs per group:
                                                                 min =           1
                                                                 avg =         1.9
                                                                 max =           2

                                                   Wald chi2(3)      =       14.30
Log likelihood = -95.634505                        Prob > chi2       =      0.0025

------------------------------------------------------------------------------
        pain |      Coef.   Std. Err.      z    P>|z|     [95% Conf. Interval]
-------------+----------------------------------------------------------------
   treatment |  -.3224315   .1310258    -2.46   0.014    -.5792373   -.0656258
    sequence |   .0461549   .1914969     0.24   0.810    -.3291721    .4214819
             |
   treatment#|
    sequence |  -.0304802    .180218    -0.17   0.866    -.3837009    .3227406
             |
       _cons |   2.096702   .1405916    14.91   0.000     1.821148    2.372257
------------------------------------------------------------------------------

------------------------------------------------------------------------------
  Random-effects Parameters  |   Estimate   Std. Err.    [95% Conf. Interval]
-----------------------------+------------------------------------------------
patient: Identity            |
                 var(_cons)  |   .2776214   .0766168     .1616375    .4768304
-----------------------------+------------------------------------------------
               var(Residual) |   .1957202   .0400325     .1310785    .2922401
------------------------------------------------------------------------------
LR test vs. linear model: chibar2(01) = 20.30          Prob >= chibar2 = 0.0000
```

Output 5.4 Results of a longitudinal mixed model analysis to estimate the treatment effect in the example cross-over trial including the interaction between treatment and sequence

To analyze the possible effect modifying effect of the sequence, sequence and the interaction between sequence and treatment are added to the model. Output 5.4 shows the results of this analysis.

The most interesting part of Output 5.4 is the interaction between treatment and sequence. The regression coefficient of the interaction reflects the difference in treatment effect between the two sequences. The regression coefficient is very low (-0.0304802), so the difference in treatment between the two sequences is ignorable. This conclusion is also supported by the p-value of the interaction (0.866), which is far from significance.

The conclusion of the analysis including sequence as an effect modifier is, however, not surprising. From Table 5.3 it can be seen that the pain values after the second phase of the trial were not different for both sequences. So the higher starting point for the patients of the intervention group who started the cross-over trial with the treatment condition did not result in a different pain level after the second phase of the cross-over trial.

In the example cross-over trial, a baseline measurement is performed for each of the conditions (see Table 5.1). Therefore, it is possible to add the baseline value to the model. It is, however, questionable whether an adjustment for the baseline value is necessary in a cross-over trial. Because each patient receives both the intervention and control condition, the estimated treatment effect cannot be biased by differences in the baseline value between the intervention and control condition. Besides that, the differences in the measurement before the second phase are not totally caused by chance. In the example cross-over trial, for instance, part of the difference is probably caused by the fact that part of the population received the intervention in the first phase of the trial.

5.3 Alternative Analyses

Although an adjustment for the baseline value is not necessary in a cross-over trial, in the example trial for each phase (both the control and treatment phase), a baseline measurement was performed. Therefore, another possibility to estimate the treatment effect is to analyze the differences in the changes in the outcome from baseline to follow-up between the treatment and the control phase. Table 5.4 shows the data structure needed to perform this analysis.

Output 5.5 shows the result of the analysis of changes performed on the example dataset.

In the first part of Output 5.5, it can be seen that there are 101 changes analyzed in 54 patients. This is exactly the same as the number of observations analyzed in the earlier analysis reported in Sect. 5.2. In the second part of the output, the regression coefficient for the treatment variable (-0.2869975) indicates the difference in outcome between the treatment phase and the control phase for each patient. The outcome variable in this analysis is the change score from baseline to follow-up. Because in a cross-over trial each patient receives both the treatment and the control condition, the change scores within one patient can be correlated. Therefore, a random intercept on patient level was added to the model. In the last part of Output 5.5, the random intercept variance is reported and also (in the lowest line of the output) the result of the likelihood ratio test with which the model without a random intercept is compared to the model with a random intercept. The p-value of this likelihood ratio test equals 0.4822 and is therefore not statistically significant. Basically this means that the correlations between the change scores within the patient are relatively low, and, therefore, it is not really necessary to add a random intercept to the model. This is different from the analyses performed in Sect. 5.2, where the likelihood ratio test comparing the model with a random intercept and the

Table 5.4 Data structure needed to perform an analysis of changes in cross-over trials

id	Change	Time	Intervention	Sequence[a]
1	$Y_{t1} - Y_{t01}$	0	1	1
1	$Y_{t2} - Y_{t02}$	1	0	1
2	$Y_{t1} - Y_{t01}$	0	0	0
2	$Y_{t2} - Y_{t02}$	1	1	0

[a]Sequence 1 indicates that a subject started with the intervention condition followed by the control condition

```
Mixed-effects ML regression                      Number of obs     =         101
Group variable: patient                          Number of groups  =          54

                                                 Obs per group:
                                                              min =           1
                                                              avg =         1.9
                                                              max =           2

                                                 Wald chi2(1)      =        4.48
Log likelihood = -104.85985                      Prob > chi2       =      0.0343

------------------------------------------------------------------------------
      change |      Coef.   Std. Err.      z    P>|z|     [95% Conf. Interval]
-------------+----------------------------------------------------------------
   treatment |  -.2869975    .135607    -2.12   0.034    -.5527824   -.0212127
       _cons |   -.352951   .0956914    -3.69   0.000    -.5405027   -.1653993
------------------------------------------------------------------------------


------------------------------------------------------------------------------
  Random-effects Parameters  |   Estimate   Std. Err.     [95% Conf. Interval]
-----------------------------+------------------------------------------------
patient: Identity            |
                  var(_cons) |   .0029177   .0654232     2.39e-22     3.56e+16
-----------------------------+------------------------------------------------
                var(Residual)|   .4640822    .092174     .3144364     .684947
------------------------------------------------------------------------------
LR test vs. linear model: chibar2(01) = 2.0e-03        Prob >= chibar2 = 0.4822
```

Output 5.5 Results of the comparison of changes from baseline to follow-up in the example cross-over trial

model without a random intercept was highly significant (see Output 5.1). This seems a bit strange, because basically the analyses are based on the same data. However, it is often the case that in a dataset where the observed values are highly correlated, the change scores are not correlated at all. It should be noted that although statistically it is not necessary to add a random intercept for patient to the model, in practice this random intercept mostly stays in the model. This has more or less a theoretical reason, because not taking into account the fact that the different measurements are performed on the same subject/patient is theoretically wrong (see also Sect. 4.4). Because of this low correlation, it is also not necessary to evaluate the necessity of adding a random slope for treatment to the model, although, theoretically, in a cross-over trial, it is possible to add a random slope to the model, because the treatment variable is time-dependent. The estimated treatment effect based on the change scores (-0.287) was slightly lower than the estimated treatment effect based on the analysis performed on the observed values (-0.339). The standard error of the estimate, however, was much lower in the analysis performed on the observed values (0.136 versus 0.090), which indicates that the effect estimation performed on the observed values is more efficient than the effect estimation based on the individual change scores.

Comparable to the analysis performed in Sect. 5.2, also when the change scores are analyzed, the next step in the analysis can (must) be the analyses of the possible effect modifying effect of sequence. This has to be done in order to detect a possible carry-over effect.

```
Mixed-effects ML regression              Number of obs       =       101
Group variable: patient                  Number of groups    =        54

                                         Obs per group:
                                                       min =         1
                                                       avg =       1.9
                                                       max =         2

                                         Wald chi2(3)        =      6.09
Log likelihood = -104.08283              Prob > chi2         =    0.1072

-------------------------------------------------------------------------
      change |     Coef.   Std. Err.      z    P>|z|    [95% Conf. Interval]
-------------+-----------------------------------------------------------
   treatment | -.1721739   .1959296   -0.88   0.380   -.5561888    .211841
    sequence | -.0093168   .1908339   -0.05   0.961   -.3833443   .3647107
             |
  treatment#|
    sequence | -.2306832   .2705669   -0.85   0.394   -.7609846   .2996181
             |
       _cons | -.3478261      .1414   -2.46   0.014    -.624965  -.0706872
-------------------------------------------------------------------------


-------------------------------------------------------------------------
  Random-effects Parameters |   Estimate   Std. Err.    [95% Conf. Interval]
----------------------------+--------------------------------------------
patient: Identity           |
               var(_cons) |   3.59e-10   1.86e-09    1.43e-14   9.03e-06
----------------------------+--------------------------------------------
             var(Residual) |    .459861    .0647114    .3490165   .6059088
-------------------------------------------------------------------------
LR test vs. linear model: chibar2(01) = 0.00          Prob >= chibar2 = 1.0000
```

Output 5.6 Results of the comparison of changes between baseline and follow-up in the example cross-over trial including the interaction between treatment and sequence

To analyze the possible effect modifying effect of the sequence, sequence and the interaction between treatment and sequence are added to the model. Output 5.6 shows the results of this analysis.

The most interesting part of Output 5.6 is the interaction between treatment and sequence. The regression coefficient of the interaction reflects the difference in treatment effect between the two sequences. In contrast to the analysis of the observed values after treatment or control including the interaction between treatment and sequence, the regression coefficient for the interaction is quite high (−0.2306832). It should be realized that the regression coefficient for treatment in Output 5.7 reflects the treatment effect for patients with sequence equals zero. So, for the patients who receive first the control condition and then the treatment condition, the treatment effect equals −0.1721739. For the patients who receive first the treatment condition and then the control condition, the treatment effect can be calculated by adding up the regression coefficient for treatment and the regression coefficient for the interaction between treatment and sequence (−0,1,721,739 + −0.2306832). The treatment for these patients is, therefore, much higher (−0.40285710), which indicates a carry-over effect. It should be noted that although the treatment effects for the different sequences are highly different, the *p*-value of the interaction between treatment and sequence is far from significance

```
Mixed-effects ML regression                    Number of obs     =        47

                                               Wald chi2(0)      =         .
Log likelihood = -44.846725                    Prob > chi2       =         .
------------------------------------------------------------------------------
  difference |      Coef.   Std. Err.      z    P>|z|     [95% Conf. Interval]
-------------+----------------------------------------------------------------
       _cons |  -.3404255   .0916456    -3.71   0.000    -.5200475   -.1608035
------------------------------------------------------------------------------


------------------------------------------------------------------------------
  Random-effects Parameters   |   Estimate   Std. Err.    [95% Conf. Interval]
------------------------------+-----------------------------------------------
              var(Residual)   |   .3947488   .0814305      .2634701    .5914394
------------------------------------------------------------------------------
```

Output 5.7 Result of the analysis comparing differences between the treatment and control phase in the example cross-over trial

Table 5.5 Data structure needed to perform an analysis of the difference between intervention and control phase in a cross-over trial

id	Difference	Sequence[a]
1	$Y_{t1} - Y_{t2}$	1
2	$Y_{t2} - Y_{t1}$	0

[a]Sequence 1 indicates that a subject started with the intervention condition followed by the control condition

(0.394), which indicates that the difference between the treatment effects for the different sequences is not statistically significant. That this relative big difference between the two treatment effects is not significant has to do with the relatively small sample size in this example cross-over trial.

A second alternative way to estimate the treatment effect in a cross-over trial is to analyze the differences between the outcome measurement after the treatment phase and the outcome measurement after the control phase. Table 5.5 shows the data structure needed to perform this analysis.

In this analysis, the longitudinal nature of the data (i.e., two measurements for each patient) is reduced to cross-sectional, i.e., only one difference score for each patient. Because there is only one outcome for each patient, there is no need to adjust for the correlated observations within the patient, i.e., there is no need to add a random intercept to the mixed model analysis. Furthermore, it should be noted that an intercept only model should be used to estimate the effect of the treatment. Output 5.7 shows the result of this analysis.

From the first part of Output 5.7, it can be seen that there are 47 difference scores analyzed. Because the outcome is the difference between the treatment and the control phase, only the patients with a measurement after both the treatment and control phase are included in the analysis. Furthermore, from the random part of the model, it can be seen that there is only residual variance and no random intercept variance. Again, that is because there is only one outcome for each patient, so there are no correlated observations within the patient. From the fixed part of the model, the effect estimate can be derived. In this particular situation, the intercept value (−0.3404255) indicates the average difference in pain between the intervention phase and the control phase. The 95% confidence interval around this difference ranges between −0.5200475 and − 0.1608035 and the corresponding p-value <0.001.

In the analysis comparing individual differences between the treatment and control phase, it is not possible to add the interaction between treatment and sequence to the model. The only possibility to estimate the different treatment effects for the different sequences is to perform two stratified analyses.

Comparing the results reported in Output 5.7 with the other results, it can be seen that the effect estimates obtained from the analysis of the individual differences between the treatment and control phase are almost the same as the ones reported in the analysis with the observed values. The small differences between the effect estimates are due to the few patients with either only a measurement after the intervention phase or only a measurement after the control phase. These patients were not included in the analysis of the differences between treatment and control phase but are included in the analysis with the observed values.

Chapter 6
Analysis of Data from a Stepped Wedge Trial

6.1 Introduction

The stepped wedge trial design is a one-way cross-over trial in which several arms start with the intervention at different time points (see Fig. 6.1). The starting point of the intervention is randomized, and although this randomization can be on the subject level, it is mostly on a cluster level, such as hospitals, nursery homes, or schools. Although there is some debate about the usefulness of a stepped wedge trial (Kotz et al., 2012), it is increasingly popular as an alternative for the regular RCT.

Besides the discussion about the usefulness of a stepped wedge trial design (a discussion which will not be covered in this book), there is also much confusion about the way data from a stepped wedged trial should be analyzed. In a systematic review, Brown and Lilford (2006) mentioned that "no two studies use the same method in analyzing data", while Mdege et al. (2011) concluded that there was a huge variation in statistical methods used, varying from simple cross-sectional statistical methods, such as t-tests or Mann-Whitney U tests to more complicated methods, such as mixed models. It is clear that there is no consensus regarding the way the data from stepped wedge trials should be analyzed.

Most stepped wedge trial designs are longitudinal in nature. This means that the same group of subjects is followed over time and the different clusters receive the intervention at different points in time. There are also stepped wedge trial designs that are cross-sectional regarding the subjects. In those stepped wedge trial designs at each interval, new subjects are included, and depending on the timing and the cluster in which they are randomized, they receive either the intervention or the control condition. It is also possible that the stepped wedge trial design is a combination of both. The focus of this chapter is on stepped wedge trial designs that are longitudinal in nature.

The most important issue to be considered in the analysis of data from a longitudinal stepped wedge trial is the one-way cross-over nature of the design. Because of that, the effect of the intervention can be measured partly within the

© The Author(s), under exclusive license to Springer Nature Switzerland AG 2021 73
J. W. R. Twisk, *Analysis of Data from Randomized Controlled Trials*,
https://doi.org/10.1007/978-3-030-81865-4_6

arm	time			
	baseline	2	3	4
1	0	X	X	X
2	0	0	X	X
3	0	0	0	X

0 = control; X = intervention

Fig. 6.1 Schematic illustration of a stepped wedge trial design with three arms and four repeated measurements

subject (each subject moves at a certain point in time from the control condition to the intervention condition) and partly between the subjects (at a certain point in time, the intervention group can be compared to the control group). Ideally, these two aspects of the intervention effect should be combined in one analysis. Because of this, it is necessary that data from a stepped wedge trial are analyzed with a method that is capable to combine these effects, i.e., a mixed model analysis. Because of this, in the next part of the chapter, only variations of mixed model analysis will be considered as appropriate ways to analyze data from stepped wedge trials.

Besides the combination of the within and between-subject effects, in the analysis of data from a stepped wedge trial, also the time variable can play an important role. In a regular RCT, adjusting for the time variable is not interesting, because the control and the intervention group are measured at the same time points, i.e., the intervention variable is time-independent (see Sect. 3.7), and, therefore, adjustment for time cannot influence the estimated intervention effect. In a stepped wedge trial, this is different, because all (clusters of) subjects start with the intervention at different time points and the effects of the intervention are also measured at different time points. Therefore, the intervention variable becomes time-dependent, and, therefore, time can influence the estimated intervention effect. Finally, it should be evaluated whether or not an adjustment for baseline differences in the outcome variable should be made. In Chaps. 2 and 3, it was already discussed that an adjustment for the baseline value is necessary in order to adjust for regression to the mean. It is, however, questionable, whether an adjustment for the baseline values is also necessary in a stepped wedge trial. Especially, because part of the stepped wedge trial is basically a cross-over trial and in Chap. 5, it was already explained why an adjustment for the baseline value in a cross-over trial is not really necessary (see Sect. 5.2). In the remaining part of this chapter, several methods will be discussed that can be used to analyze data from a stepped wedge trial.

6.2 Example Dataset

The first example dataset is based on data from the ACT trial (Muntinga et al., 2012) in which primary care practices in the intervention group delivered care according to a new method, whereas practices in the control group delivered usual care. The cluster stepped wedge trial was conducted among 35 primary care practices in the Netherlands, and outcome measurements were administered at baseline and at 6, 12, 18, and 24 months. The primary outcome of the study was quality of life as measured by the 12-item Short Form questionnaire (SF-12). Figure 6.2 shows the schematic illustration of the stepped wedge example trial, and Table 6.1 shows the descriptive information.

The descriptive information clearly shows that there is a slight increase in quality of life over time, which seems to be irrespective whether the arm receives the intervention or not.

6.3 Statistical Methods

6.3.1 Comparing Intervention and Control Measurements

The most simple way to analyze the data from a stepped wedge trial is to compare all intervention measurements with all control measurements (see Fig. 6.3 and Eq. 6.1).

	time				
arm	baseline	2	3	4	5
1	0	X	X	X	X
2	0	0	X	X	X
3	0	0	0	X	X
4	0	0	0	0	X

0 = control; X = intervention

Fig. 6.2 Schematic illustration of the ACT trial

Table 6.1 Mean quality of life and standard deviation (between brackets) for the different arms at the different time points

	Time				
Arm	Baseline	2	3	4	5
1	49.1 (11.5)	50.7 (10.9)	50.6 (10.4)	52.1 (10.4)	52.8 (10.2)
2	50.2 (9.4)	49.7 (11.2)	52.9 (9.1)	52.4 (9.4)	52.9 (9.8)
3	50.3 (9.7)	49.5 (10.6)	52.5 (9.2)	51.4 (10.7)	53.1 (10.0)
4	50.8 (10.6)	51.9 (9.8)	53.7 (10.0)	53.8 (10.2)	54.5 (9.0)

	time				
arm	baseline	2	3	4	5
1	0	X	X	X	X
2	0	0	X	X	X
3	0	0	0	X	X
4	0	0	0	0	X

0 = control; X = intervention

Fig. 6.3 Illustration of method 1; all intervention measurements are compared with all control measurements

$$Y_t = \beta_0 + \beta_1 X \tag{6.1}$$

where Y_t = outcome measured at all measurements, X = intervention variable, and β_1 = overall intervention effect.

With this approach the intervention variable is a time-dependent dichotomous variable. The estimated effect of the intervention reveals the difference between all the measurements after an intervention period and all the measurements after a control period. Because the intervention effect is reflected in one number, this method does not provide an answer to the question whether a long-term exposure to the intervention is different from a short-term exposure. The possibility to make that distinction is basically one of the key features of using a stepped wedge design.

In the example stepped wedge trial, the use of a mixed model analysis is not only necessary to adjust for the correlated observations of the repeated measures within the subject but also to adjust for the correlated observations of the subjects within the primary care practice. The data has, therefore, three levels; repeated observations are clustered within the subject, and subjects are clustered within the primary care practices. Output 6.1 shows the result of the analysis comparing all intervention measurements with all control measurements.

Like any other mixed model analysis, Output 6.1 contains three parts. In the first part it can be seen that a three-level structure is used. There are 1 to 5 repeated measures clustered within 1126 subjects which are clustered within 35 practices. The second part contains the fixed part of the model in which the regression coefficient for the intervention variable is given. This coefficient (1.776702) indicates the overall difference in quality of life on average over time between all intervention measurements and all control measurements. This difference has a 95% confidence interval ranging from 1.2792 to 2.274204 and a corresponding p-value <0.001. The last part of the output shows the random part of the model, which contains the random intercept variance on the subject level (54.31918) and the random intercept variance on the practice level (1.534278). These numbers indicate that the correlation between the repeated observations within the subject is much higher than the correlation between the subject observations within the practice. This is, of course, as expected. It should be noted that in this example a priori a random intercept for

```
Mixed-effects ML regression                    Number of obs      =      4,273

-------------------------------------------------------------------
               |   No. of      Observations per Group
Group Variable |   Groups    Minimum   Average   Maximum
---------------+---------------------------------------------------
      practice |       35         11     122.1       328
            id |    1,126          1       3.8         5
-------------------------------------------------------------------

                                               Wald chi2(1)       =      48.99
Log likelihood = -15385.204                    Prob > chi2        =     0.0000

-------------------------------------------------------------------------------
          Qol |     Coef.   Std. Err.       z    P>|z|     [95% Conf. Interval]
--------------+----------------------------------------------------------------
 intervention |  1.776702   .2538322     7.00    0.000      1.2792     2.274204
        _cons |  50.27717   .3587895   140.13    0.000     49.57396    50.98039
-------------------------------------------------------------------------------


-------------------------------------------------------------------------------
 Random-effects Parameters    |    Estimate   Std. Err.     [95% Conf. Interval]
------------------------------+------------------------------------------------
practice: Identity            |
                  var(_cons)  |    1.534278   .8994289       .486307    4.840585
------------------------------+------------------------------------------------
id: Identity                  |
                  var(_cons)  |   54.31918    3.050589      48.65746    60.63971
------------------------------+------------------------------------------------
                var(Residual) |   52.27385    1.314673      49.75961    54.91512
-------------------------------------------------------------------------------
LR test vs. linear model: chi2(2) = 1333.42             Prob > chi2 = 0.0000
```

Output 6.1 Results of the mixed model analysis to compare all intervention measurements with all control measurements

practice level is modeled. A random intercept on the subject level is always necessary because otherwise the longitudinal nature of the data is ignored, which is theoretically wrong (see also Sect. 4.4). For the random intercept on practice level, the situation is slightly different, because it is not obligatory to add a random intercept on practice level to the model. Basically the necessity of a random intercept on practice level could be evaluated with likelihood ratio test (see Chap. 4). However, in the present example, it was decided to add a random intercept on practice level a priori to the model.

The highly significant positive regression coefficient suggests a relatively strong intervention effect. However, in the descriptive information (Table 6.1), it was seen that there was a gradual increase in quality of life over time irrespective of the intervention. Because the number of intervention observations in a stepped wedge trial increases over time (see Figs. 6.1 and 6.2), the estimated intervention effect can be highly biased by the effect of time. Therefore, in the next step of the analysis, time is added to the model as a covariate (Eq. 6.2):

$$Y_t = \beta_0 + \beta_1 X + \beta_2 time_1 + \beta_3 time_2 + \beta_4 time_3 + \beta_5 time_4 \qquad (6.2)$$

```
Mixed-effects ML regression                     Number of obs     =      4,273

-----------------------------------------------------------------
              |    No. of      Observations per Group
Group Variable |    Groups    Minimum    Average    Maximum
--------------+--------------------------------------------------
     practice |        35         11      122.1        328
           id |      1,126         1        3.8          5
-----------------------------------------------------------------

                                                Wald chi2(5)      =      85.88
Log likelihood = -15366.821                     Prob > chi2       =     0.0000

-------------------------------------------------------------------------------
         Qol |     Coef.    Std. Err.      z     P>|z|    [95% Conf. Interval]
-------------+-----------------------------------------------------------------
intervention |   .0539694   .3975063     0.14    0.892    -.7251287    .8330675
             |
        time |
           2 |   .3389319   .3685123     0.92    0.358    -.383339    1.061203
           3 |   1.69668    .4184155     4.06    0.000    .8766002    2.516759
           4 |   2.019246   .4752602     4.25    0.000    1.087754    2.950739
           5 |   2.782769   .5395577     5.16    0.000    1.725256    3.840283
             |
       _cons |   49.92907   .3591174   139.03    0.000    49.22522   50.63293
-------------------------------------------------------------------------------

-------------------------------------------------------------------------------
Random-effects Parameters  |   Estimate   Std. Err.    [95% Conf. Interval]
---------------------------+---------------------------------------------------
practice: Identity         |
             var(_cons)    |   .9050629   .7364453    .1836793    4.459614
---------------------------+---------------------------------------------------
id: Identity               |
             var(_cons)    |   54.13491   3.035528    48.50066    60.42368
---------------------------+---------------------------------------------------
          var(Residual)    |   51.84829   1.304312    49.35388    54.46876
-------------------------------------------------------------------------------
LR test vs. linear model: chi2(2) = 1319.60              Prob > chi2 = 0.0000
```

Output 6.2 Results of the mixed model analysis to compare all intervention measurements with all control measurements adjusted for time

where Y_t = outcome measured at all measurements, X = intervention variable, β_1 = overall intervention effect, and $time_1$, $time_2$, $time_3$, and $time_4$ = dummy variables for the different time points.

Output 6.2 shows the result of this analysis.

From the fixed part of Output 6.2, it can be seen that time is added to the model. The four regression coefficients for the time dummy variables indicate the difference in the outcome quality of life between that particular time point and the reference time point, which is the first measurement (i.e., the baseline measurement). Based on the regression coefficients of the time dummy variables, it can be seen that there is an increase in quality of life over time. It can be concluded that the estimated development over time is independent of the intervention, because the intervention variable is part of the model. The most striking difference in the results shown in Output 6.1 and in Output 6.2 is the regression coefficient for the intervention variable. Adjusting for time, the regression coefficient for the intervention variable reduced from 1.776702 to 0.0539694, with a 95% confidence interval ranging from −0.7251287 to 0.8330675, and a corresponding p-value of 0.892. So, the conclusion based on the results reported in Output 6.2 are totally different from the ones reported in Output 6.1. Compared to the descriptive information depicted in Table 6.1, the results reported in Output 6.2 are a much better reflection of what is happening in the data. So, based on the analysis performed so far, it can be concluded that there is an increase in quality of life over time, irrespective of the intervention. This indicates that there is no actual effect of the intervention.

6.3.2 Comparing Different Arms

As has been mentioned before, with the method comparing all intervention measurements with all control measurements, no distinction can be made between possible short-term and long-term effects of the intervention. There are other methods available to analysis data from a stepped wedge trial, in which that distinction can be made. In one of those methods, the intervention variable is a time-independent categorical variable comparing the different arms with each other. Each arm is a different combination of intervention and control measurements (see Fig. 6.4 and Eq. 6.3). The general idea behind this analysis is that each arm has a different number of intervention measurements. Arm 1 has four intervention measurements, while arm 4 only has one intervention measurement:

$$Y_t = \beta_0 + \beta_1 arm_1 + \beta_2 arm_2 + \beta_3 arm_3 \qquad (6.3)$$

where Y_t = outcome measured at all measurements; arm_1, arm_2, and arm_3 = dummy variables for the different arms; and β_1, β_2, and β_3 = differences in outcome between the particular arm and the reference arm.

Output 6.3 shows the results of the analysis. In this analysis arm 4 is taken as the reference category because arm 4 has the least amount of intervention measurements.

arm	time				
	baseline	2	3	4	5
1	0	X	X	X	X
2	0	0	X	X	X
3	0	0	0	X	X
4	0	0	0	0	X

0 = control; X = intervention

Fig. 6.4 Illustration of method 2; the four arms are compared with each other

```
Mixed-effects ML regression                    Number of obs     =      4,273

------------------------------------------------------------------
              |  No. of     Observations per Group
Group Variable |  Groups   Minimum    Average    Maximum
--------------+---------------------------------------------------
     practice |      35       11       122.1        328
           id |   1,126        1         3.8          5
------------------------------------------------------------------

                                              Wald chi2(3)      =       6.21
Log likelihood = -15406.562                   Prob > chi2       =     0.1018

------------------------------------------------------------------------
        Qol |     Coef.   Std. Err.      z    P>|z|     [95% Conf. Interval]
------------+-----------------------------------------------------------
        arm |
          1 |  -1.896517   .772904    -2.45   0.014    -3.411381   -.3816531
          2 |  -1.083137   .8805944   -1.23   0.219    -2.80907     .6427965
          3 |  -1.456784   .8728086   -1.67   0.095    -3.167458    .2538894
            |
      _cons |  52.28932    .6219055   84.08   0.000    51.0704     53.50823
------------------------------------------------------------------------


------------------------------------------------------------------------
  Random-effects Parameters  |  Estimate   Std. Err.    [95% Conf. Interval]
-----------------------------+------------------------------------------
practice: Identity           |
              var(_cons)     |  .4316443   .6004566     .0282506    6.595154
-----------------------------+------------------------------------------
id: Identity                 |
              var(_cons)     |  54.67099   3.077813     48.95949   61.04879
-----------------------------+------------------------------------------
           var(Residual)     |  53.02363   1.334445     50.47163   55.70467
------------------------------------------------------------------------
LR test vs. linear model: chi2(2) = 1286.58          Prob > chi2 = 0.0000
```

Output 6.3 Results of the mixed model analysis comparing the different arms

The first part of Output 6.3 is the same as shown in the earlier outputs. The same holds for the random part of the model. The difference is found in the fixed part of the model, which now shows the regression coefficients of the dummy variables for the different arms. The regression coefficient for arm 1 (-1.896517) indicates the difference in quality of life on average over time between the subjects in arm 1 compared to the subjects in arm 4. This basically indicates that the quality of life on average over time is 1.9 points lower in the group with the most intervention measurements compared to the group with the least amount of intervention measurements. This difference has a 95% confidence interval ranging from -3.411381 to -0.3816531 and a corresponding p-value of the 0.014. The regression coefficients for the other two dummy variables indicate the differences in quality of life on average over time between arm 2 and arm 4 and between arm 3 and arm 4, respectively.

Because in this method, the intervention variable (i.e., the dummy variables representing the different arms) is a time-independent categorical variable, the analysis is comparable to the analysis of a regular RCT with a categorical intervention variable. This means, for instance, that an adjustment for time is not really

```
Mixed-effects ML regression                    Number of obs    =      3,044
Group variable: id                             Number of groups =        907

                                               Obs per group:
                                                            min =          1
                                                            avg =        3.4
                                                            max =          4

                                               Wald chi2(4)     =     484.10
Log likelihood = -10780.84                     Prob > chi2      =     0.0000

------------------------------------------------------------------------------
         Qol |    Coef.   Std. Err.      z    P>|z|    [95% Conf. Interval]
-------------+----------------------------------------------------------------
         arm |
           1 |  -.859166   .6303599    -1.36  0.173   -2.094649    .3763167
           2 | -1.054442   .721021     -1.46  0.144   -2.467617    .3587335
           3 | -1.355319   .7128403    -1.90  0.057   -2.752461    .0418219
             |
baseline_Qol |   .4776011  .0218764    21.83  0.000    .434724     .5204781
       _cons |  28.55637   1.232674    23.17  0.000   26.14037    30.97237
------------------------------------------------------------------------------


------------------------------------------------------------------------------
  Random-effects Parameters  |   Estimate   Std. Err.    [95% Conf. Interval]
-----------------------------+------------------------------------------------
id: Identity                 |
                 var(_cons)  |  30.90482    2.25667     26.78376    35.65997
-----------------------------+------------------------------------------------
               var(Residual) |  50.39718    1.537181    47.47265    53.50187
------------------------------------------------------------------------------
LR test vs. linear model: chibar2(01) = 456.05        Prob >= chibar2 = 0.0000
```

Output 6.4 Results of the mixed model analysis comparing the different arms with each other adjusted for the baseline value

necessary, because all arms are measured at the same time points. On the other hand, because the intervention variable is time-independent (i.e., there is no within-subject comparison), an adjustment for the baseline value can be performed. Because the subjects are randomized into the different arms from one (source) population, the differences in quality of life observed between the arms at baseline are due to chance and can therefore cause regression to the mean (see Sect. 2.1). From Table 6.1, it can be seen that there is a difference in baseline values between the arms, so an adjustment for the baseline quality of life can be of influence. Output 6.4 shows the result of this analysis.

First of all, it should be realized that the number of observations used in the analysis adjusted for the baseline value is much lower than the number of observations used in the analysis without adjusting for the baseline value. That has to do with the fact that in the analysis without the baseline value, the baseline value was analyzed as part of the outcome variable. In the analysis adjusted for the baseline, this is (of course) not the case. This means that the regression coefficients reported in Outputs 6.3 and 6.4 cannot be directly compared to each other. Secondly, from the output it can be seen that there is no random intercept on practice level. Due to the less number of observations used as outcome and the adjustment for the baseline value, the random intercept variance on practice level could not be estimated, and, therefore, in the analysis only an adjustment was made for the correlated repeated observations within the subject.

From the regression coefficient shown in the fixed part of the output, it can be seen that the estimated differences between the arms are still in favor of arm 4, i.e., the arm with the least amount of intervention measurements.

Because the intervention variable is a time-independent variable, which is comparable to a regular RCT, the next step in the analysis can be an analysis including time and the interaction between arm and time (Eq. 6.4):

$$
\begin{aligned}
Y_t = {} & \beta_0 + \beta_1 arm_1 + \beta_2 arm_2 + \beta_3 arm_3 + \beta_4 time_1 + \beta_5 time_2 + \beta_6 time_3 \\
& + \beta_7 arm_1 \times time_1 + \beta_8 arm_1 \times time_2 + \beta_9 arm_1 \times time_3 + \beta_{10} arm_2 \\
& \times time_1 + \beta_{11} arm_2 \times time_2 + \beta_{12} arm_3 \times time_3 + \beta_{13} arm_3 \times time_1 \\
& + \beta_{14} arm_3 \times time_2 + \beta_{15} arm_3 \times time_3
\end{aligned}
\tag{6.4}
$$

where Y_t = outcome measured at all measurements, arm_1, arm_2, and arm_3 = dummy variables for the different arms; $time_1$, $time_2$, $time_3$, and $time_4$ = dummy variables for the different time points; and β_1, β_2, and β_3 = differences in outcome between the particular arm and the reference arm at the reference time point.

In this model, the regression coefficients of the dummy variables for the different arms indicate the difference between the arms at the first measurement. In this analysis the first measurement is time point 2, because the baseline value is not used as outcome but as covariate. In Chap. 3 it was already explained that analyzing the data with different reference categories for time provide the differences between the arms at the other time points. Output 6.5 shows the results of the analysis including time and the interaction between arm and time, using the first time point as reference.

Although Output 6.5 looks a bit complicated because it contains a lot of regression coefficients, the interpretation of the output is not that difficult. The most important regression coefficients are the ones of the dummy variables for the different arms. They indicate the differences between the first three arms and arm 4 at the second time point. It can be seen that all three arms have a lower quality of life than arm 4, which is most pronounced for arm 2 and arm 3. This is rather strange because at the second time point, arm 2, arm 3, and arm 4 all received only the control condition. The difference between arm 1 (the only arm that received the intervention) and arm 4 is less pronounced (-0.3915612), but the difference is still in favor of arm 4, which is basically the control condition.

Besides reanalyzing the data with a different reference time point (which makes it possible to compare the different arms with each other at the different time points), it is also possible to reanalyze the data with a different reference category for the arms. Output 6.6 shows for instance the same results as has been reported in Output 6.5 but now with arm 3 as reference arm.

The regression coefficient for arm 1 shown in Output 6.6 (1.59631) now indicates the difference in quality of life between arm 1 and arm 3 at the second time point. Because at this time point arm 1 received the intervention and arm 3 received the

```
Mixed-effects ML regression                      Number of obs     =      3,044
Group variable: id                               Number of groups  =        907

                                                 Obs per group:
                                                              min =          1
                                                              avg =        3.4
                                                              max =          4

                                                 Wald chi2(16)     =     559.85
Log likelihood = -10745.323                      Prob > chi2       =     0.0000

------------------------------------------------------------------------------
         Qol |     Coef.   Std. Err.      z    P>|z|     [95% Conf. Interval]
-------------+----------------------------------------------------------------
         arm |
           1 |  -.3915612   .8381972    -0.47   0.640    -2.034398    1.251275
           2 |  -1.768241   .959555     -1.84   0.065    -3.648934    .1124522
           3 |  -1.987872   .9475685    -2.10   0.036    -3.845072   -.1306716
             |
        time |
           2 |   1.456071   .794816      1.83   0.067    -.1017396    3.013882
           3 |   1.725608   .796937      2.17   0.030     .1636399    3.287576
           4 |   2.209616   .8056842     2.74   0.006     .6305044    3.788728
             |
    arm#time |
         1#2 |  -1.457721   .9737942    -1.50   0.134    -3.366323    .4508803
         1#3 |  -.2791876   .9852202    -0.28   0.777    -2.210184    1.651809
         1#4 |  -.0342082   1.00356     -0.03   0.973    -2.001149    1.932732
         2#2 |   1.297795   1.11753      1.16   0.246    -.8925232    3.488114
         2#3 |   .7897539   1.134273     0.70   0.486    -1.43338     3.012887
         2#4 |   .9556261   1.143079     0.84   0.403    -1.284767    3.196019
         3#2 |   1.460865   1.103698     1.32   0.186    -.7023434    3.624073
         3#3 |   .0060439   1.112347     0.01   0.996    -2.174116    2.186204
         3#4 |   1.428965   1.144591     1.25   0.212    -.8143921    3.672323
             |
 baseline_Qol|   .4750456   .0217993    21.79   0.000     .4323197    .5177715
       _cons |   27.43689   1.306098    21.01   0.000     24.87698    29.99679
------------------------------------------------------------------------------


------------------------------------------------------------------------------
  Random-effects Parameters  |   Estimate   Std. Err.    [95% Conf. Interval]
-----------------------------+------------------------------------------------
id: Identity                 |
                 var(_cons)  |   31.02035   2.235569      26.9341    35.72654
-----------------------------+------------------------------------------------
               var(Residual) |   48.91135   1.491296      46.07409   51.92334
------------------------------------------------------------------------------
LR test vs. linear model: chibar2(01) = 476.99        Prob >= chibar2 = 0.0000
```

Output 6.5 Results of the mixed model analysis comparing the different arms with each other including time and the interaction between arm and time and adjusted for the baseline value

control condition, the positive difference between the two arms can be interpreted as a positive intervention effect. However, in the analysis reported earlier, it was obvious that there is no evidence of a positive intervention effect, so the results of the analysis should not be interpreted as a single result but should always be interpreted in light of the total picture.

```
Mixed-effects ML regression                    Number of obs      =      3,044
Group variable: id                             Number of groups   =        907

                                               Obs per group:
                                                             min =          1
                                                             avg =        3.4
                                                             max =          4

                                               Wald chi2(16)      =     559.85
Log likelihood = -10745.323                    Prob > chi2        =     0.0000

-----------------------------------------------------------------------------
       Qol |     Coef.    Std. Err.      z     P>|z|    [95% Conf. Interval]
-----------+-----------------------------------------------------------------
       arm |
         1 |   1.59631    .8215013     1.94    0.052    -.0138025    3.206423
         2 |   .2196305   .945331      0.23    0.816    -1.633184    2.072445
         4 |   1.987872   .9475685     2.10    0.036     .1306716    3.845072
           |
      time |
         2 |   2.916936   .7658105     3.81    0.000     1.415975    4.417897
         3 |   1.731652   .7760363     2.23    0.026     .2106484    3.252655
         4 |   3.638582   .813027      4.48    0.000     2.045078    5.232085
           |
  arm#time |
       1#2 |  -2.918586   .9502565    -3.07    0.002    -4.781055   -1.056118
       1#3 |  -.2852314   .9683868    -0.29    0.768    -2.183235    1.612772
       1#4 |  -1.463173   1.009441    -1.45    0.147    -3.441641    .5152939
       2#2 |  -.1630697   1.097083    -0.15    0.882    -2.313313    1.987174
       2#3 |   .78371     1.119686     0.70    0.484    -1.410833    2.978253
       2#4 |  -.4733391   1.148274    -0.41    0.680    -2.723915    1.777236
       4#2 |  -1.460865   1.103698    -1.32    0.186    -3.624073    .7023434
       4#3 |  -.0060439   1.112347    -0.01    0.996    -2.186204    2.174116
       4#4 |  -1.428965   1.144591    -1.25    0.212    -3.672323    .8143921
           |
baseline_Qol | .4750456  .0217993    21.79    0.000     .4323197    .5177715
      _cons |  25.44902   1.286175    19.79    0.000     22.92816    27.96987
-----------------------------------------------------------------------------


-----------------------------------------------------------------------------
  Random-effects Parameters |    Estimate   Std. Err.    [95% Conf. Interval]
-----------------------------+-----------------------------------------------
id: Identity                 |
               var(_cons)    |    31.02035   2.235569     26.9341     35.72654
-----------------------------+-----------------------------------------------
             var(Residual)   |    48.91135   1.491296     46.07409    51.92334
-----------------------------------------------------------------------------
LR test vs. linear model: chibar2(01) = 476.99         Prob >= chibar2 = 0.0000
```

Output 6.6 Results of the mixed model analysis comparing the different arms with each other including time and the interaction between arm and time and adjusted for the baseline value and with arm 3 as reference arm

6.3.3   Comparing Groups with a Different Number of Intervention Measurements

In the second method that is capable to make a distinction between short-term and long-term effects of the intervention, the intervention variable is a time-dependent categorical variable comparing groups with different number of intervention measurements with a group containing all the control measurements. This method is

arm	time				
	baseline	2	3	4	5
1	0	X	X	X	X
2	0	0	X	X	X
3	0	0	0	X	X
4	0	0	0	0	X

0 = control condition; X = intervention

Fig. 6.5 Illustration of method 3; groups with a different number of intervention measurements are compared with each other

basically an extension of the first method, in which the intervention group from the first method (i.e., all intervention measurements) is divided into subgroups defined according to the number of intervention measurements (see Fig. 6.5 and Eq. 6.5). The different number of intervention measurements reflects the amount of time a particular subject receives the intervention; it actually represents the length of the received intervention. The more intervention measurements, the longer the length of the received intervention:

$$Y_t = \beta_0 + \beta_1 month_1 + \beta_2 month_2 + \beta_3 month_3 + \beta_4 month_4 \qquad (6.5)$$

where Y_t = outcome measured at all measurements; $month_1$, $month_2$, $month_3$, and $month_4$ = dummy variables for the groups with a different number of intervention measurement (i.e., the amount on months the group received the intervention); and β_1, β_2, β_3, and β_4 = differences in outcome between the particular group and the group containing all control measurements.

In the example trial, the measurements are performed after 6, 12, 18, and 24 months. So, for instance, the first dummy variable equals 6 months and indicates one intervention measurement. This group includes the second measurement for the subjects randomized in arm 1, the third measurement for the subjects randomized in arm 2, the fourth measurement for the subjects randomized in arm 3, and the fifth and last measurement for the subjects randomized in arm 4. It should be noted that in this example the length (in months) of the received intervention corresponds totally with the number of intervention measurements. This has to do with the fact that in this example the repeated measurements are performed with equally spaced time intervals. When the time intervals between the repeated measurements were not equal, the number of intervention measurements will not correspond totally with the length of the received intervention. Output 6.7 shows the results of the analysis.

From Output 6.7 it can be seen that again a three-level structure is used. The repeated observations are clustered within subjects, and the subjects are clustered within practices. In the random part of the model, the random intercept variances of both levels are shown. In the fixed part of the model, there are four regression coefficients for the four dummy variables representing the different number of

```
Mixed-effects ML regression                    Number of obs    =    4,273

------------------------------------------------------------------
            |   No. of      Observations per Group
Group Variable |   Groups    Minimum    Average    Maximum
------------+-----------------------------------------------------
   practice |      35          11       122.1        328
         id |   1,126           1         3.8          5
------------------------------------------------------------------

                                         Wald chi2(4)     =      63.44
Log likelihood = -15378.243              Prob > chi2      =     0.0000

------------------------------------------------------------------
       Qol |    Coef.    Std. Err.     z    P>|z|    [95% Conf. Interval]
-----------+------------------------------------------------------
    months |
         6 |   1.42575   .3090841    4.61   0.000    .8199557    2.031543
        12 |   1.568444  .3578261    4.38   0.000    .8671177     2.26977
        18 |   2.532432  .4189374    6.04   0.000    1.711329    3.353534
        24 |   3.119227  .522857     5.97   0.000    2.094446    4.144008
           |
     _cons |  50.24086   .3669065  136.93   0.000   49.52173    50.95998
------------------------------------------------------------------


------------------------------------------------------------------
Random-effects Parameters |  Estimate   Std. Err.    [95% Conf. Interval]
--------------------------+---------------------------------------
practice: Identity        |
             var(_cons)   |  1.717695   .9506425    .5805724    5.082013
--------------------------+---------------------------------------
id: Identity              |
             var(_cons)   |  54.3509    3.049103    48.6916     60.66796
--------------------------+---------------------------------------
           var(Residual)  |  52.02991   1.308495    49.52749    54.65877
------------------------------------------------------------------
LR test vs. linear model: chi2(2) = 1344.24          Prob > chi2 = 0.0000
```

Output 6.7 Results of mixed model analysis comparing groups with a different number of intervention measurements

intervention measurements. The regression coefficient for 6 months (1.42575) indicates the difference between all measurements after 6 months of intervention and all control measurements. The regression coefficient for 12 months (1.568444) indicates the difference between all measurements after 12 months of intervention and all control measurements, etc. Based on the results shown in Output 6.7, it can be concluded that the longer the intervention is applied, the higher the quality of life of the subjects, which indicates a positive intervention effect. However, also in this analysis, the differences between the groups with a different number of intervention measurements are probably biased by time. This is because the measurements with a longer intervention time are also the measurements at the end of the study, and because there is gradual increase in quality of life over time (irrespective of the intervention), the estimated effects can be biased. Therefore, the model is extended with time and the interaction between months and time (see Eq. 6.6):

$$Y_t = \beta_0 + \beta_1 month_1 + \beta_2 month_2 + \beta_3 month_3 + \beta_4 month_4 + \beta_5 time_1$$
$$+ \beta_6 time_2 + \beta_7 time_3 + \beta_8 time_4 \qquad (6.6)$$

where Y_t = outcome measured at all measurements; $month_1$, $month_2$, $month_3$, and $month_4$ = dummy variables for the groups with a different number of intervention measurement (i.e., the amount on months the group received the intervention); $time_1$, $time_2$, $time_3$, and $time_4$ = dummy variables for the different time points; and β_1, β_2, β_3, and β_4 = differences in outcome between the particular group and the group containing all control measurements.

Output 6.8 shows the result of this analysis.

In the fixed part of Output 6.8, it is obvious that the regression coefficients for the groups representing the number of intervention measurements were highly reduced when time was added to the model. Basically, the same happened in the first analysis in which all intervention measurements were compared with all control measurements (method 1). Only the regression coefficient for 6 months of intervention remained positive (0.2151271), but the difference with the group containing all control measurements is rather small and far from significant ($p = 0.613$). The regression coefficients for 12, 18, and 24 months in intervention even became negative after the adjustment for time. So, based on the analysis performed with this third method, the conclusion is the same. There is an increase in quality of life over time, which is independent of the intervention.

6.3.4 Comparing Transitions

The last method to analyze data from a stepped wedge trial is slightly different from the first three methods, in such a way that instead of the observed values of the outcome variables at the different time points, the changes in the outcome variable between subsequent measurements are analyzed. These transitions are then compared between three transition groups: (1) subjects moving from control condition to control condition, (2) subjects moving from control condition to intervention condition, and (3) subjects moving from intervention condition to intervention condition (see Fig. 6.6 and Eq. 6.7):

$$Y_t - Y_{t-1} = \beta_0 + \beta_1 group_1 + \beta_2 group_2 \qquad (6.7)$$

where Y_t = outcome measured at all measurements after the baseline measurement, Y_{t-1} = outcome measured at all measurements besides at the last time point, $group_1$ and $group_2$ = dummy variables for the transition groups, and β_1 and β_2 = differences in outcome between the transition groups.

```
Mixed-effects ML regression                    Number of obs    =      4,273

-----------------------------------------------------------------
                |  No. of       Observations per Group
 Group Variable |  Groups    Minimum    Average    Maximum
----------------+------------------------------------------------
       practice |      35         11      122.1        328
             id |   1,126          1        3.8          5
-----------------------------------------------------------------

                                              Wald chi2(8)     =      89.70
Log likelihood = -15364.958                   Prob > chi2      =     0.0000

-----------------------------------------------------------------------------
          Qol |     Coef.    Std. Err.      z    P>|z|    [95% Conf. Interval]
--------------+--------------------------------------------------------------
       months |
            6 |   .2151271   .4248811     0.51   0.613    -.6176246   1.047879
           12 |  -.5992817   .5543283    -1.08   0.280    -1.685745    .4871819
           18 |  -.0387032   .7210509    -0.05   0.957    -1.451937   1.374531
           24 |  -.2266728   .9592996    -0.24   0.813    -2.106866    1.65352
              |
         time |
            2 |   .2779046   .3729712     0.75   0.456    -.4531055   1.008915
            3 |   1.921638   .4444068     4.32   0.000     1.050617   2.792659
            4 |   2.151057   .5571196     3.86   0.000     1.059123   3.242991
            5 |    3.00574     .73183     4.11   0.000      1.57138   4.440101
              |
        _cons |   49.92417   .3554418   140.46   0.000     49.22751   50.62082
-----------------------------------------------------------------------------


-----------------------------------------------------------------------------
 Random-effects Parameters   |   Estimate   Std. Err.    [95% Conf. Interval]
-----------------------------+-----------------------------------------------
practice: Identity           |
                var(_cons)   |   .8278039   .7217963     .1498752   4.572199
-----------------------------+-----------------------------------------------
id: Identity                 |
                var(_cons)   |   54.11493   3.034186     48.48315   60.40089
-----------------------------+-----------------------------------------------
              var(Residual)  |    51.809    1.30355      49.31606   54.42795
-----------------------------------------------------------------------------
LR test vs. linear model: chi2(2) = 1316.45             Prob > chi2 = 0.0000
```

Output 6.8 Results of the mixed model analysis comparing groups with a different number of intervention measurements adjusted for time

arm	time				
	baseline	2	3	4	5
1	0	X	X	X	X
2	0	0	X	X	X
3	0	0	0	X	X
4	0	0	0	0	X

0 = control; X = intervention

Fig. 6.6 Illustration of method 4; groups with a different transition are compared with each other

```
Mixed-effects ML regression                      Number of obs    =      3,009

-------------------------------------------------------------
                     |   No. of        Observations per Group
  Group Variable |    Groups    Minimum    Average    Maximum
-----------------+-------------------------------------------
       practice |        35          7       86.0        227
             id |       936          1        3.2          4
-------------------------------------------------------------

                                              Wald chi2(2)    =        1.09
Log likelihood = -11130.634                   Prob > chi2     =      0.5805

-------------------------------------------------------------------------
  Qol_change |     Coef.    Std. Err.       z    P>|z|     [95% Conf. Interval]
-------------+-----------------------------------------------------------
       group |
           1 |   .4825637    .4683142     1.03    0.303    -.4353153    1.400443
           2 |    .156589    .4177686     0.37    0.708    -.6622225    .9754004
             |
       _cons |   .3290253    .3125189     1.05    0.292    -.2835004    .9415511
-------------------------------------------------------------------------


-------------------------------------------------------------------------
  Random-effects Parameters  |   Estimate   Std. Err.     [95% Conf. Interval]
-----------------------------+-------------------------------------------
practice: Identity           |
                 var(_cons)  |   1.34e-15    1.12e-14     1.06e-22    1.70e-08
-----------------------------+-------------------------------------------
id: Identity                 |
                 var(_cons)  |   7.91e-18    1.29e-17     3.27e-19    1.91e-16
-----------------------------+-------------------------------------------
              var(Residual)  |   95.61703    3.135745     89.66444    101.9648
-------------------------------------------------------------------------
LR test vs. linear model: chi2(2) = 0.00                Prob > chi2 = 1.0000
```

Output 6.9 Results of the mixed model analysis comparing the different transition groups regarding the change in quality of life

The general idea of this analysis is that when there is a short-term effect of the intervention, the transition from the control condition to the intervention condition directly has an effect on the outcome, while a transition from the intervention condition to the intervention condition would not has an effect on the outcome. When there is a short-term and long-term effect of the intervention, both transitions would lead to an effect on the outcome, and when there is only a long-term effect of the intervention, the biggest effect will be observed after a transition from the intervention condition to the intervention condition.

Output 6.9 shows the results of the analysis with the group who moved from the control condition to the control condition as the reference group.

Output 6.9 looks similar to the other three-level mixed model analyses performed so far. The most interesting part is the fixed part of the model which contains the regression coefficients. The regression coefficient for group 1 (0.4825637) indicates the difference in the change in quality of life between the transition from control to intervention compared to the transition from control to control. The positive sign of the regression coefficient indicates that there is a stronger increase in quality of life when a subject goes from the control to the intervention condition than when a subject stays in the control condition. The regression coefficient for group 2 (0.156589) indicates the difference in change in quality of life for the transition from intervention to intervention compared to the transition from control to control. So, both regression coefficients are positive, but the corresponding p-values are far above the significance level.

It should also be noted that the random intercept variances shown in the random part of the model are very low. This holds for the random intercept variance on the subject level as well as for the random intercept variance on the practice level. This may look strange, because in the earlier analyses, the random intercept variances (especially the one on the subject level) were quite high. However, the analysis performed in this method uses the change in quality of life as outcome, while all other analyses used the observed quality of life as outcome. It is important to realize that changes between subsequent measurements are often not correlated within the same subject even though the observed values themselves are highly correlated within the same subject (see also Sect. 5.3). Because the change scores between subsequent measurements are not correlated to each other, the random intercept variances reduce to almost zero. When there is no random intercept variance on both levels, the three-level mixed model analysis could also been analyzed with a regular linear regression analysis. The results would have been exactly the same.

Also for the comparison of the transition groups, it should be noted that the transitions to the intervention condition for subjects in different arms occur at different time points. So, when there is an increase or decrease in the outcome over time irrespective of the intervention, also the effect estimates of the transition analysis are biased. Therefore, in the next step in the analysis, time is added to the model (see Eq. 6.8).

$$Y_t - Y_{t-1} = \beta_0 + \beta_1 group_1 + \beta_2 group_2 + \beta_3 time_1 + \beta_4 time_2 + \beta_4 time_3 \quad (6.8)$$

where Y_t = outcome measured at all measurements after the baseline; Y_{t-1} = outcome measured at all measurements besides at the last time point; $group_1$ and $group_2$ = dummy variables for the transition groups; $time_1$, $time_2$, and $time_3$ = dummy variables for the time point where the particular change in the outcome is calculated; and β_1 and β_2 = differences in outcome between the transition groups.

Because the changes between two subsequent measurements are used as outcome, there are four time point represented by three dummy variables. Output 6.10 shows the result of the analysis.

From Output 6.10 it can be seen that the regression coefficients for the transition groups are not much different from the regression coefficients shown in Output 6.9. This indicates that the increase in quality of life over time independent of the intervention does not bias the effect estimates of the transition groups. The

```
Mixed-effects ML regression                    Number of obs       =      3,009

-----------------------------------------------------------------
             |   No. of        Observations per Group
Group Variable |   Groups   Minimum    Average    Maximum
---------------+-------------------------------------------------
      practice |       35         7       86.0        227
            id |      936         1        3.2          4
-----------------------------------------------------------------

                                             Wald chi2(5)      =       8.49
Log likelihood = -11126.938                  Prob > chi2       =     0.1311

-------------------------------------------------------------------------------
  Qol_change |     Coef.   Std. Err.      z    P>|z|     [95% Conf. Interval]
-------------+-----------------------------------------------------------------
       group |
          1  |  .4635782   .4809831     0.96   0.335    -.4791314    1.406288
          2  | -.1984712   .5253161    -0.38   0.706    -1.228072    .8311295
             |
        time |
          2  |  1.360418   .5172283     2.63   0.009     .3466691    2.374167
          3  |  .5012802   .5649396     0.89   0.375    -.605981    1.608542
          4  |  .8623655   .6287426     1.37   0.170    -.3699473    2.094678
             |
       _cons | -.1777504   .3824041    -0.46   0.642    -.9272488    .5717479
-------------------------------------------------------------------------------


-------------------------------------------------------------------------------
 Random-effects Parameters  |  Estimate   Std. Err.    [95% Conf. Interval]
----------------------------+--------------------------------------------------
practice: Identity          |
                 var(_cons) |  5.75e-14   5.28e-13     8.78e-22    3.76e-06
----------------------------+--------------------------------------------------
id: Identity                |
                 var(_cons) |  2.38e-17   4.07e-17     8.23e-19    6.85e-16
----------------------------+--------------------------------------------------
               var(Residual) |  95.3824   2.745905     90.14954    100.919
-------------------------------------------------------------------------------
LR test vs. linear model: chi2(2) = 0.00           Prob > chi2 = 1.0000
```

Output 6.10 Results of the mixed model analysis comparing the different transition groups regarding the change in quality of life adjusted for time

conclusion of the transition analysis is, however, the same as the other analysis, i.e., there is no actual effect of the intervention.

6.4   A Second Example

6.4.1   Introduction

Because of the complexity of the analysis of a stepped wedge trial, in this section, a second example will be discussed. In the second example a cluster stepped wedge RCT is performed within pain clinics of 17 hospitals which were randomly divided over five arms. Six measurements took place: one baseline measurement and a measurement every 4 weeks during a period of twenty weeks. After each

arm	time					
	baseline	2	3	4	5	6
1	0	X	X	X	X	X
2	0	0	X	X	X	X
3	0	0	0	X	X	X
4	0	0	0	0	X	X
5	0	0	0	0	0	X

0 = control; X = intervention

Fig. 6.7 Schematic illustration of the second example cluster stepped wedge RCT

Table 6.2 Mean pain scores and standard deviation (between brackets) for the different arms at the different time points

Arm	Time					
	Baseline	2	3	4	5	6
1	3.8 (0.4)	3.7 (0.3)	3.7 (0.4)	3.6 (0.4)	3.6 (0.3)	3.5 (0.3)
2	3.8 (0.3)	3.9 (0.3)	3.8 (0.3)	3.7 (0.3)	3.7 (0.3)	3.6 (0.3)
3	3.9 (0.3)	3.9 (0.3)	3.9 (0.3)	3.8 (0.3)	3.8 (0.3)	3.6 (0.3)
4	3.9 (0.4)	3.9 (0.3)	3.8 (0.3)	4.0 (0.3)	4.0 (0.3)	3.8 (0.3)
5	3.9 (0.4)	4.1 (0.4)	4.0 (0.4)	4.0 (0.4)	4.1 (0.4)	4.2 (0.4)

measurement cycle, a new arm started the intervention. The aim of the intervention was to reduce pain for patients suffering from chronic pain. The outcome variable pain was continuous and ranged between 1 and 5, where 5 indicates the most pain. Figure 6.7 shows the schematic illustration of the stepped wedge example RCT and Table 6.2 shows the descriptive information.

From the descriptive information shown in Table 6.2, it can be seen that there seems to be a small decrease in pain over time and that this decrease is partly caused by the intervention. For this example, the same analyses were performed as for the first example dataset.

6.4.2   Comparing Intervention and Control Measurements

In the first method, all intervention measurements were compared with all control measurements. The intervention variable is therefore a time-dependent dichotomous variable (see Sect. 6.3.1). Output 6.11 shows the result of the analysis.

From Output 6.11 it can be seen that the regression coefficient for the intervention is -0.0969672. This number indicates the difference in pain between all intervention measurements and all control measurements on average over time. The 95%

```
Mixed-effects ML regression                      Number of obs      =      2,284

-------------------------------------------------------------
              |   No. of        Observations per Group
Group Variable |    Groups    Minimum    Average    Maximum
---------------+---------------------------------------------
     hospital |       17          92      134.4        174
      patient |      655           1        3.5          6
-------------------------------------------------------------

                                              Wald chi2(1)       =      63.71
Log likelihood = -380.50452                   Prob > chi2        =     0.0000

------------------------------------------------------------------------------
        pain |     Coef.    Std. Err.      z     P>|z|    [95% Conf. Interval]
-------------+----------------------------------------------------------------
intervention |  -.0969672   .0121489    -7.98    0.000    -.1207786   -.0731558
       _cons |   3.873502   .0357191   108.44    0.000     3.803493    3.94351
------------------------------------------------------------------------------


------------------------------------------------------------------------------
 Random-effects Parameters   |   Estimate   Std. Err.    [95% Conf. Interval]
-----------------------------+------------------------------------------------
hospital: Identity           |
                 var(_cons)  |   .018894    .0073033     .0088573     .040304
-----------------------------+------------------------------------------------
patient: Identity            |
                 var(_cons)  |   .0630357   .0046555     .0545409    .0728537
-----------------------------+------------------------------------------------
             var(Residual)   |   .0515109   .0017997     .0481017    .0551618
------------------------------------------------------------------------------
LR test vs. linear model: chi2(2) = 1002.23        Prob > chi2 = 0.0000
```

Output 6.11 Results of the mixed model analysis to compare all intervention measurements with all control measurements

confidence interval around this difference ranges from -0.1207786 to -0.0731558, and the corresponding p-value is <0.001.

In the first part of Output 6.11, it can be seen that a three-level mixed model analysis is performed in which the repeated measurements are clustered within patients, and the patients are clustered within hospitals. In the third part of het output, the random intercept variances are given. As in the first example, it can be seen that the random intercept variance on the patient level is much higher than the random intercept variance on the hospital level, indicating that the correlation between the repeated observations within the patient is stronger than the correlation between the patient observations within the hospital.

As in the first example, the next step in the analysis is an adjustment for time. Therefore, five time dummy variables are added to the model (see Sect. 6.3.1). Output 6.12 shows the result of this analysis.

In Output 6.12 it can be seen that the adjustment for time attenuated the regression coefficient for the intervention variable. The difference between the intervention measurements and control measurements was -0.0969672 without adjustment for time and -0.0433674 with adjustment for time. The 95% confidence interval around this difference ranges from -0.0786624 to -0.0080723, and the corresponding p-value is 0.016. So, the estimated intervention effect is partly caused

```
Mixed-effects ML regression                        Number of obs      =      2,284

---------------------------------------------------------------------
              |   No. of         Observations per Group
Group Variable |   Groups    Minimum    Average    Maximum
--------------+------------------------------------------------------
     hospital |      17          92       134.4        174
      patient |     655           1         3.5          6
---------------------------------------------------------------------

                                              Wald chi2(6)       =     107.91
Log likelihood = -359.09313                   Prob > chi2        =     0.0000


---------------------------------------------------------------------------
        pain |     Coef.    Std. Err.      z     P>|z|     [95% Conf. Interval]
-------------+-------------------------------------------------------------
intervention |  -.0433674    .018008    -2.41    0.016    -.0786624   -.0080723
             |
        time |
           2 |   .0295252   .0168384     1.75    0.080    -.0034775    .0625279
           3 |  -.0053885   .0186689    -0.29    0.773    -.0419788    .0312018
           4 |  -.0201423   .0209057    -0.96    0.335    -.0611168    .0208322
           5 |  -.0178463   .0227192    -0.79    0.432    -.062375     .0266824
           6 |  -.1068593   .0252082    -4.24    0.000    -.1562664   -.0574522
             |
       _cons |  3.866999   .0390327    99.07    0.000     3.790496    3.943501
---------------------------------------------------------------------------


---------------------------------------------------------------------------
 Random-effects Parameters  |   Estimate   Std. Err.     [95% Conf. Interval]
----------------------------+----------------------------------------------
hospital: Identity          |
              var(_cons)    |   .0217089   .0082969      .010264     .0459154
----------------------------+----------------------------------------------
patient: Identity           |
              var(_cons)    |   .0627926   .0046138      .0543707    .0725191
----------------------------+----------------------------------------------
            var(Residual)   |   .0502808   .0017562      .0469538    .0538436
---------------------------------------------------------------------------

LR test vs. linear model: chi2(2) = 1025.87               Prob > chi2 = 0.0000
```

Output 6.12 Results of the mixed model analysis to compare all intervention measurements with all control measurements adjusted for time

by a regular decrease in pain over time, but even in an analysis adjusting for time, there is still a significant intervention effect.

6.4.3   Comparing Different Arms

In the second method, the different arms are compared with each other. In this method the intervention variable is a categorical time-independent variable (see Sect. 6.3.2). Note that in this analysis, arm 1 is used as reference arm. In arm 1, the patients receive the most intervention measurements (see Fig. 6.7). Output 6.13 shows the results of the analysis.

From Output 6.13 it can be seen that the regression coefficients for the different arms are increasing with the number of control measurements that were performed

```
Mixed-effects ML regression                          Number of obs      =      2,284

-----------------------------------------------------------------
                   |   No. of         Observations per Group
  Group Variable   |   Groups    Minimum    Average    Maximum
-------------------+---------------------------------------------
        hospital   |      17          92       134.4        174
         patient   |     655           1         3.5          6
-----------------------------------------------------------------

                                                   Wald chi2(4)       =       48.81
Log likelihood = -400.19401                        Prob > chi2        =      0.0000

-----------------------------------------------------------------------------
        pain  |    Coef.    Std. Err.      z     P>|z|    [95% Conf. Interval]
--------------+--------------------------------------------------------------
         arm  |
           2  |  .1132414   .0625588    1.81    0.070   -.0093717     .2358544
           3  |  .1629385   .0631854    2.58    0.010    .0390974     .2867796
           4  |  .2825011   .0679791    4.16    0.000    .1492645     .4157377
           5  |  .4341882   .0681326    6.37    0.000    .3006507     .5677257
              |
       _cons  | 3.634641    .0478109   76.02    0.000   3.540934     3.728349
-----------------------------------------------------------------------------


-----------------------------------------------------------------------------
  Random-effects Parameters  |   Estimate   Std. Err.    [95% Conf. Interval]
-----------------------------+-----------------------------------------------
hospital: Identity           |
                var(_cons)   |   .0045976   .0023868     .0016621     .0127181
-----------------------------+-----------------------------------------------
patient: Identity            |
                var(_cons)   |   .0639661   .0047409     .0553175     .0739669
-----------------------------+-----------------------------------------------
              var(Residual)  |   .0530188   .0018508     .0495125     .0567732
-----------------------------------------------------------------------------
LR test vs. linear model: chi2(2) = 861.58              Prob > chi2 = 0.0000
```

Output 6.13 Results of the mixed model analysis comparing the different arms

within a particular arm. The regression coefficient for arm 2 (0.1132414) indicates the difference in pain on average over time between arm 2 (for which the intervention started at the third measurement) and arm 1 (for which the intervention started at the second measurement). In the same way, the regression coefficient for arm 5 (0.4341882) indicates the difference in pain on average over time between arm 5 (for which the intervention started at the last measurement) and arm 1. So, in general, less intervention measurements lead to a higher average pain score indicating a possible intervention effect. Because the intervention variable is a time-independent variable, there is no need to adjust the analysis for time. Again, this has to do with the fact that all arms were measured at the same time points. To illustrate that time does not influence the effect estimates, Output 6.14 shows the results of the analysis comparing different arms with each other adjusted for time.

As expected, adding time to the model has no influence on the estimated regression coefficients for the different arms. There is only a very small difference which is caused by a different amount of missing data in the different arms. When there were no missing observations (i.e., when a complete case analysis was

```
Mixed-effects ML regression                    Number of obs    =      2,284

-----------------------------------------------------------------
                   |   No. of        Observations per Group
 Group Variable    |   Groups    Minimum    Average    Maximum
-------------------+---------------------------------------------
         hospital  |       17         92      134.4        174
          patient  |      655          1        3.5          6
-----------------------------------------------------------------

                                               Wald chi2(9)     =     152.31
 Log likelihood = -350.33496                   Prob > chi2      =     0.0000

------------------------------------------------------------------------------
        pain  |     Coef.    Std. Err.      z     P>|z|    [95% Conf. Interval]
--------------+---------------------------------------------------------------
         arm  |
           2  |   .1141864   .0617175     1.85    0.064    -.0067777    .2351506
           3  |   .1666091   .0623411     2.67    0.008     .0444228    .2887954
           4  |   .2739778   .0670735     4.08    0.000     .1425161    .4054394
           5  |   .4362146   .0672252     6.49    0.000     .3044556    .5679735
              |
        time  |
           2  |   .0218232   .0165462     1.32    0.187    -.0106067    .0542532
           3  |  -.0240369   .0170076    -1.41    0.158    -.0573711    .0092973
           4  |  -.0489568   .0171699    -2.85    0.004    -.0826092   -.0153044
           5  |   -.051918   .0178049    -2.92    0.004     -.086815    -.017021
           6  |  -.1488141     .01827    -8.15    0.000    -.1846227   -.1130055
              |
       _cons  |   3.675178   .0484137    75.91    0.000     3.580289    3.770067
------------------------------------------------------------------------------


------------------------------------------------------------------------------
  Random-effects Parameters  |   Estimate   Std. Err.    [95% Conf. Interval]
-----------------------------+------------------------------------------------
hospital: Identity           |
                var(_cons)   |   .0044692   .0023249     .0016122     .012389
-----------------------------+------------------------------------------------
patient: Identity            |
                var(_cons)   |   .0628882   .0046213     .0544527    .0726306
-----------------------------+------------------------------------------------
              var(Residual)  |   .0503792   .0017582     .0470484    .0539458
------------------------------------------------------------------------------
LR test vs. linear model: chi2(2) = 896.32           Prob > chi2 = 0.0000
```

Output 6.14 Results of the mixed model analysis comparing the different arms with each other adjusted for time

performed), the regression coefficients (i.e., effect estimates) would have been exactly the same in analyses with and without adjusting for time.

More interesting than the adjustment for time is the adjustment for the baseline value of the outcome variable. It has been mentioned before that, at baseline, the arms are randomized from the same (source) population and that, therefore, the differences at baseline between the arms are due to chance (similar to a regular RCT). Therefore, the analysis comparing the different arms with each other can be adjusted for the baseline value of the outcome variable. Output 6.15 shows the results of this analysis.

In Output 6.15 it can be seen that the adjustment for the baseline value of the outcome variable pain does not have a huge influence on the effect estimates.

```
Mixed-effects ML regression                        Number of obs    =    1,242

-----------------------------------------------------------------
                  |   No. of         Observations per Group
 Group Variable   |   Groups    Minimum    Average    Maximum
------------------+----------------------------------------------
       hospital   |      17          50       73.1         99
        patient   |     338           1        3.7          5
-----------------------------------------------------------------

                                                   Wald chi2(5)     =     295.97
Log likelihood = -97.920511                        Prob > chi2      =     0.0000

-----------------------------------------------------------------------------
          pain |    Coef.    Std. Err.      z     P>|z|     [95% Conf. Interval]
---------------+-------------------------------------------------------------
           arm |
             2 |  .1587935   .0557077     2.85    0.004     .0496083    .2679787
             3 |   .214467   .0561238     3.82    0.000     .1044665    .3244676
             4 |  .2492776   .0611588     4.08    0.000     .1294086    .3691465
             5 |  .3960308   .0596372     6.64    0.000      .279144    .5129176
               |
 baseline_pain |  .5701048   .0367985    15.49    0.000      .497981    .6422286
         _cons |  1.433223   .1479601     9.69    0.000     1.143226    1.723219
-----------------------------------------------------------------------------


-----------------------------------------------------------------------------
  Random-effects Parameters  |  Estimate   Std. Err.     [95% Conf. Interval]
-----------------------------+-----------------------------------------------
hospital: Identity           |
                 var(_cons)  |  .0029684    .001887       .0008539    .0103186
-----------------------------+-----------------------------------------------
patient: Identity            |
                 var(_cons)  |   .031498   .0036839       .0250455    .0396128
-----------------------------+-----------------------------------------------
              var(Residual)  |   .049553    .002305       .0452351     .054283
-----------------------------------------------------------------------------
LR test vs. linear model: chi2(2) = 257.41            Prob > chi2 = 0.0000
```

Output 6.15 Results of the mixed model analysis comparing the different arms adjusted for the baseline value

However, the comparison between the effect estimates reported in Output 6.13 cannot be compared directly with the effect estimates reported in Output 6.15, because the population used in both analyses is different. In Output 6.13, all measurements are used as outcome, while with the adjustment for baseline, the baseline value itself is not used as outcome anymore but only as covariate. Therefore, the number of observations reduces from 2284 to 1242. Nevertheless, based on the descriptive information shown in Table 6.2, it could be seen that there is not much difference between the baseline values of the different arms, so it is expected that an adjustment for these differences would not make a big difference.

```
Mixed-effects ML regression                 Number of obs      =      2,284

-------------------------------------------------------------------
                    |    No. of        Observations per Group
  Group Variable    |    Groups    Minimum   Average   Maximum
--------------------+----------------------------------------------
        hospital    |       17         92      134.4       174
         patient    |      655          1        3.5         6
-------------------------------------------------------------------

                                            Wald chi2(5)       =     217.14
Log likelihood = -309.12794                 Prob > chi2        =     0.0000

-------------------------------------------------------------------------
          pain |     Coef.    Std. Err.      z     P>|z|    [95% Conf. Interval]
---------------+---------------------------------------------------------
time_in_in~n   |
            4  |  -.0193173   .0144921    -1.33   0.183    -.0477213    .0090868
            8  |  -.1043944   .0161749    -6.45   0.000    -.1360965   -.0726923
           12  |   -.180519   .0177033   -10.20   0.000    -.2152168   -.1458212
           16  |  -.2336987    .022192   -10.53   0.000    -.2771942   -.1902031
           20  |  -.3268278   .0333784    -9.79   0.000    -.3922483   -.2614074
               |
        _cons  |   3.887455   .0314771   123.50   0.000     3.825761    3.949149
-------------------------------------------------------------------------


-------------------------------------------------------------------------
  Random-effects Parameters    |   Estimate   Std. Err.    [95% Conf. Interval]
-------------------------------+-----------------------------------------
hospital: Identity             |
                 var(_cons)    |   .0141339   .005649      .0064574    .0309361
-------------------------------+-----------------------------------------
patient: Identity              |
                 var(_cons)    |   .0617757   .0044916     .0535708    .0712373
-------------------------------+-----------------------------------------
               var(Residual)   |   .0479233   .0016723     .0447552    .0513156
-------------------------------------------------------------------------
LR test vs. linear model: chi2(2) = 1008.10          Prob > chi2 = 0.0000
```

Output 6.16 Results of the mixed model analysis comparing groups with a different number of intervention measurements

6.4.4 Comparing Groups with a Different Number of Intervention Measurements

As has been mentioned before, the method comparing groups with a different number of intervention measurements, i.e., comparing patients which received the intervention for a different amount of time, is basically an extension of the method in which all intervention measurements were compared with all control measurements. The extension indicates that the population who received the intervention is divided into subgroups with a different number of intervention measurements (i.e., in subgroups with a different length of the received intervention). These subgroups are compared with all control measurements (see Sect. 6.3.3). Output 6.16 shows the result of this analysis.

From Output 6.16 it can be seen that the regression coefficients for the groups who received the intervention for a longer period of time are negative, so these groups have lower average pain values. For instance, the group of patients who

```
Mixed-effects ML regression                         Number of obs    =      2,284

----------------------------------------------------------
                 |   No. of       Observations per Group
 Group Variable  |   Groups    Minimum   Average   Maximum
-----------------+----------------------------------------
       hospital  |      17        92       134.4      174
        patient  |     655         1         3.5        6
----------------------------------------------------------

                                              Wald chi2(10)    =     285.86
Log likelihood = -281.36078                   Prob > chi2      =     0.0000

--------------------------------------------------------------------------------
        pain |    Coef.    Std. Err.      z     P>|z|    [95% Conf. Interval]
-------------+------------------------------------------------------------------
time_in_in~n |
          4  |  -.0906178   .0186635    -4.86   0.000    -.1271976   -.0540381
          8  |  -.2177845   .0238673    -9.12   0.000    -.2645635   -.1710056
         12  |  -.3483987   .0305074   -11.42   0.000    -.4081922   -.2886052
         16  |  -.4542614   .0393044   -11.56   0.000    -.5312965   -.3772263
         20  |  -.5790237   .0531956   -10.88   0.000    -.6832852   -.4747622
             |
        time |
          2  |   .036623    .0162624     2.25   0.024     .0047493    .0684966
          3  |   .0372376   .0182671     2.04   0.041     .0014346    .0730405
          4  |   .0872006   .0216369     4.03   0.000     .044793     .1296082
          5  |   .1880473   .0268359     7.01   0.000     .1354499    .2406447
          6  |   .2057461   .0343515     5.99   0.000     .1384184    .2730737
             |
       _cons |  3.863957    .0271897   142.11   0.000     3.810667    3.917248
--------------------------------------------------------------------------------


--------------------------------------------------------------------------------
 Random-effects Parameters  |   Estimate   Std. Err.    [95% Conf. Interval]
----------------------------+---------------------------------------------------
hospital: Identity          |
               var(_cons)   |   .0085787   .003764      .0036303    .0202721
----------------------------+---------------------------------------------------
patient: Identity           |
               var(_cons)   |   .0620688   .0044772     .0538858    .0714945
----------------------------+---------------------------------------------------
            var(Residual)   |   .0465729   .0016249     .0434945    .0498691
--------------------------------------------------------------------------------
LR test vs. linear model: chi2(2) = 982.33             Prob > chi2 = 0.0000
```

Output 6.17 Result of the mixed model analysis comparing groups with a different number of intervention measurements adjusted for time

received the intervention for 20 weeks (i.e., the patients with five intervention measurements) has a 0.3268278 lower average pain score compared with all control measurements. It can also be seen that this difference is highly significant ($p < 0.001$). For the group of patients who received the intervention for only 4 weeks (i.e., the patients with only one intervention measurement) on the other hand, a regression coefficient of -0.0193173 was found, which indicates that this group of patients has on average a 0.019 lower pain score than all control measurements. The 95% confidence interval around this difference ranges from -0.0477213 to 0.00908680 and the corresponding p-value $= 0.183$. As has been mentioned before, the measurements taken on the patients who received the intervention for the longest time are also the measurements taken in the last part of the study. It is, therefore, possible that the effect estimates reported in Output 6.15 are biased by time. Therefore, in the next step of the analysis, time is added to the model (see Sect. 6.3.3). Output 6.17 shows the result of this analysis.

Comparing the effect estimates based on a model without the adjustment for time with the effect estimates based on a model with the adjustment for time, it can be seen that the effect estimates for the latter are stronger. So, not taking time into account leads to underestimated effect estimates. This is a bit unexpected, because in the first method, where all intervention measurements were compared with all control measurements, an adjustment for time resulted in a lower effect estimate. From Output 6.17 it can further be seen that in the model including the intervention variable comparing different number of the intervention measurements and time, the regression coefficients for time are all positive, which indicates that there is increase in pain over time when the intervention variable comparing the different number of intervention measurements is taken into account. In Output 6.12, where all intervention measurements were compared with all control measurements, the regression coefficients for time were mostly negative, which indicates a decreasing trend in pain when the overall intervention variable is taken into account. In Table 6.2 it can be seen that there is an increase in pain over time for the control measurements, while there is a decrease in pain over time for the intervention measurements, trends that are better captured with the analyses comparing the groups with a different number of intervention measurements. It should further be noted that the results of the analysis adjusted for time must be interpreted with some caution, because the intervention variable and the time variable are highly correlated. Especially the much higher standard errors of the effect estimates in the analysis adjusted for time are a result of this high correlation. Furthermore, the high correlation can also lead to slightly overestimated effect estimates.

6.4.5   Comparing Transitions

The last method used to estimate treatment effects in a stepped wedge trial was the transition method (method 4). In this method the changes in pain were compared between three transition groups: patients moving from the control condition to the control condition, patients moving from the control condition to the intervention condition, and patients moving from the intervention condition to the intervention condition (see Sect. 6.3.4). Output 6.18 shows the result of the analysis with the group who moved from the control condition to the control condition as the reference group.

From Output 6.18 it can be seen that the regression coefficient for the transition groups are both negative, which indicates that there is a decrease in pain for the transition from control to intervention as well as the transition from intervention to intervention (compared to the transition from control to control). It can, furthermore, be seen that the regression coefficient for the intervention to intervention transition is bigger than the regression coefficient for the control to intervention transition. So,

```
Mixed-effects ML regression                    Number of obs    =      1,615

-------------------------------------------------------------
             |    No. of      Observations per Group
Group Variable |    Groups    Minimum    Average    Maximum
---------------+---------------------------------------------
    hospital |       17         58        95.0        119
     patient |      512          1         3.2          5
-------------------------------------------------------------

                                         Wald chi2(2)     =        51.20
Log likelihood =  -274.6862              Prob > chi2      =       0.0000

---------------------------------------------------------------------------
change_pain |    Coef.    Std. Err.      z     P>|z|    [95% Conf. Interval]
------------+--------------------------------------------------------------
      group |
          1 |  -.0966816  .0202765    -4.77   0.000   -.1364229   -.0569403
          2 |  -.1099994  .0160826    -6.84   0.000   -.1415208   -.0784781
            |
      _cons |   .0372727  .0117521     3.17   0.002    .014239     .0603065
---------------------------------------------------------------------------


---------------------------------------------------------------------------
  Random-effects Parameters  |  Estimate  Std. Err.    [95% Conf. Interval]
-----------------------------+---------------------------------------------
hospital: Identity           |
                 var(_cons)  |  .0000789  .0003519    1.26e-08    .4933406
-----------------------------+---------------------------------------------
patient: Identity            |
                 var(_cons)  |  2.75e-20  5.78e-20    4.46e-22    1.70e-18
-----------------------------+---------------------------------------------
               var(Residual) |  .0821979  .0029105    .0766868    .0881049
---------------------------------------------------------------------------
LR test vs. linear model: chi2(2) = 0.06             Prob > chi2 = 0.9722
```

Output 6.18 Results of the mixed model analysis comparing the different transition groups regarding the change in pain

the decrease in pain is more pronounced for the transition from intervention to intervention than for the transition from control to intervention. This finding leads more or less to the same conclusion as the finding of stronger effect estimates for patients who received the intervention for a longer period of time.

Because the different transitions take place at different time points for the different patients, it makes sense to adjust the transition analysis for time (see Sect. 6.3.4). Output 6.19 shows the result of this analysis.

From Output 6.19 it can be seen that the adjustment for time did not have a strong influence on the regression coefficients for the two transition groups. Both remain negative, with a slightly stronger effect for the intervention to intervention transition than for the control to intervention transition. Both effect estimates also remain highly significant.

Overall, based on the results of the different analyses, it can be concluded that (1) the intervention has a positive effect on pain and (2) the longer the intervention is applied, the stronger the effect.

```
Mixed-effects ML regression                      Number of obs      =      1,615

--------------------------------------------------------------------
              |    No. of      · Observations per Group
Group Variable |    Groups    Minimum    Average    Maximum
--------------+-----------------------------------------------------
     hospital |        17         58       95.0        119
           id |       512          1        3.2          5
--------------------------------------------------------------------

                                                 Wald chi2(6)       =      72.20
Log likelihood = -264.92693                      Prob > chi2        =     0.0000

--------------------------------------------------------------------------------
 change_pain |     Coef.    Std. Err.      z     P>|z|     [95% Conf. Interval]
-------------+------------------------------------------------------------------
       group |
           1 |  -.0948282    .0211855    -4.48   0.000    -.1363511    -.0533054
           2 |  -.1212356    .0215042    -5.64   0.000     -.163383    -.0790881
             |
        time |
           2 |  -.0318211    .0227036    -1.40   0.161    -.0763194     .0126773
           3 |   .0154293    .0243615     0.63   0.527    -.0323185     .063177
           4 |   .0568136    .0268563     2.12   0.034     .0041762     .109451
           5 |  -.0268648    .0286009    -0.94   0.348    -.0829216     .029192
             |
        _cons |   .0391941    .0160865     2.44   0.015     .0076651     .0707231
--------------------------------------------------------------------------------


--------------------------------------------------------------------------------
 Random-effects Parameters  |   Estimate    Std. Err.     [95% Conf. Interval]
----------------------------+---------------------------------------------------
hospital: Identity          |
               var(_cons)   |   .0000472    .0003377      3.80e-11     58.58411
----------------------------+---------------------------------------------------
id: Identity                |
               var(_cons)   |   2.28e-20    4.92e-20      3.35e-22     1.55e-18
----------------------------+---------------------------------------------------
             var(Residual)  |   .0812391    .0028767      .075792      .0870776
--------------------------------------------------------------------------------
LR test vs. linear model: chi2(2) = 0.02                   Prob > chi2 = 0.9896
```

Output 6.19 Results of the mixed model analysis comparing the different transition groups regarding the change in pain adjusted for time

6.5   Comments

It should be realized that the different methods used in this chapter analyze different aspects of the intervention effect in a (cluster) stepped wedge trial. With the first method in which all intervention measurements were compared with all control measurements, information about the length of the intervention is not taken into account. The methods comparing the different arms and comparing the different number of intervention measurements on the other hand try to estimate the effect of the length of the intervention. Although the purpose of the two methods is comparable, the results were quite different. The results obtained from the analysis comparing different arms can be interpreted as the average difference between the arms with different intervention durations. In fact these differences indicate the between-subject part of the intervention effect. The results obtained from the method comparing groups with a different number of intervention measurements reveal a more direct effect of the different intervention durations and indicate both the between and within-subject part of the intervention effect. Although this is an advantage, this method has also a (small) disadvantage, i.e., the reduction of the number of subjects with a longer duration of the intervention. This reduces the power of the analysis and makes the method more vulnerable for random fluctuations. The method, in which the changes between subsequent measurements were compared between the different transition groups, captures mostly the within-subject part of the intervention effect (Twisk, 2013; Twisk et al., 2016).

6.5.1 Adjustment for Time

Hussey and Hughes (2007) claim that effect estimates derived from a stepped wedge trial are biased when time is not included in the model. This makes sense when there is either an increase or a decrease over time in the outcome variable independent of the intervention. This is different from a regular RCT in which an adjustment for time is not necessary. Because in a regular RCT the intervention and control groups are measured at the same time points, time is not related to the intervention variable. Based on the definition of confounding (i.e., a possible confounder must be related to both the outcome variable and the independent variable), time cannot be a confounder in a regular RCT. In a stepped wedge trial design, the situation is different because the intervention variable is related to time. When time increases, the number of patients receiving the intervention increases. So when time is also associated with the outcome variable (i.e., when there is either a decrease or increase over time), time can be a confounder. The influence of time on the estimation of the effect of the intervention was nicely illustrated in the first example. The descriptive information (see Table 6.1) showed an increase over time in the whole population, irrespective of the fact whether the patient receives the intervention or not. Because at the end of the study there are more subjects in the intervention group (due to the stepped wedge trial design), this increase over time is wrongly allocated to the intervention when time is not taken into account. Adjusting for time led to a huge decrease in the estimated intervention effect. However, when the randomization arms are compared with each other, an adjustment for time is not necessary. This is due to the fact that belonging to a particular arm is not related to time, and therefore time cannot be a confounder (comparable to a regular RCT). The small differences observed in the second example dataset between the analysis of the arms with or without an adjustment for time are due to an increase in missing values over time and the selectiveness of the missing data. In a full dataset (i.e., without any missing data), the results of the analysis comparing the different arms with each other would be exactly the same with or without an adjustment for time. Also in the transition method, an adjustment for time makes sense, because in this method the independent variable (i.e., the transition group) is also related to time.

Although the adjustment for time makes sense in the methods in which the intervention variable is related to time, one should be careful with the interpretation of the results. In the method comparing all intervention measurements with all control measurements, for instance, at the first measurement, all subjects receive the control condition, while at the last measurement, all subjects receive the intervention. When an adjustment for time is performed in the analysis, basically the first and last measurement are ignored, and the intervention effect is only estimated over the in-between measurements, which is not correct. Basically the same holds for the method in which subjects with different lengths of the intervention are compared with each other. In this method, especially the estimation of the intervention effect for the group with the longest length of the intervention is slightly unreliable. This is because this group is only measured at the last follow-up measurement, while there is no control condition at the last measurement. In the analysis adjusted for time, this leads to a sort of "empty cell" problem, which leads to a less reliable result. This was also reflected in the higher standard errors of the effect estimates when the analyses were adjusted for time (see Sects. 6.3.3 and 6.4.4).

6.5.2   Adjustment for the Baseline Value

In a regular RCT, an adjustment for baseline differences is performed to adjust for possible regression to the mean. This is necessary because the two groups to be compared are taken from the same (source) population, and the differences observed at baseline are due to chance. When the differences at baseline are not taken into account, it can lead to either an over- or underestimation of the intervention effect (see Chaps. 2 and 3). Within a stepped wedge trial, basically the same arguments can be used. It should, therefore, be considered whether or not the intervention variable is analyzed as a time-dependent or time-independent variable. In method 2 in which the arms were compared with each other, the intervention variable (i.e., the different arms) is analyzed as time-independent. Then, basically the same rules can be applied as for a regular RCT. In fact, the arms are randomized, and the differences between the arms at baseline are due to chance. Therefore, in the method comparing different arms, an adjustment for the baseline value of the outcome variable makes sense. In the other three methods, the intervention variable is analyzed as a time-dependent variable. So, in general by using these methods, an adjustment for the baseline value of the outcome is not really necessary (Twisk et al., 2016).

6.5.3   Recommendation

It is important to realize that the analyses of data from a stepped wedge trial are not as straightforward as for the analysis of data from a regular RCT. Different methods reveal different aspects of a possible intervention effect, and therefore the choice of a

Table 6.3 Considerations for the different methods used to analyze data from a stepped wedge trial

Pros and cons	Method 1	Method 2	Method 3	Method 4
Between-subject and/or within-subject effects	Both	Only between	Both	Mostly within
Is it necessary to adjust for time?	Yes	No	Yes	Yes
Possibility to analyze influence of length of intervention	No	Yes	Yes	No
Is it necessary to adjust for the baseline value?	As in a regular RCT	As in a regular RCT	As in a regular RCT	As in a regular RCT
Possibility to detect delay in treatment effect	No	Yes	Yes	Yes (partly)

Method 1 = comparing all intervention measurements with all control measurements; method 2 = comparing different arms; method 3 = comparing groups with a different number of intervention measurements; method 4 = comparing transitions

method partly depends on the specific research question. So, unfortunately, it is not possible to give a straightforward advice which of the methods should be used. Table 6.3 summarizes the pros and cons of the different methods discussed in this chapter. In general, the results obtained from the method comparing groups with a different number of intervention measurements probably provide the best estimation of the intervention effect, because this method combines the between-subject and within-subject effect of the intervention. The most stable results are obtained from the method comparing the different arms, especially because the results are not influenced by time. The disadvantage, however, is that with this method, only the between-subject part of the intervention effect is estimated.

Chapter 7
Analysis of Data from an *N*-of-1 Trial

7.1 Introduction

Basically, an *n*-of-1 trial can be seen as a series of cross-over trials performed in the same subject. And although *n*-of-1 trials can be performed in different settings, they are mostly applied in the medical field. The general idea behind an *n*-of-1 trial (which is also known as an individual patient trial or a single case RCT) is to find the best treatment or intervention for an individual patient. This idea fits perfectly within the framework of personalized medicine, which is a popular novel approach in the treatment and care of individual patients. The series of cross-over trials can be done with the same treatment, but it is more common to perform the *n*-of-1 trial with different treatments or different dose of medicine, etc. (see Fig. 7.1).

Probably the best way to analyze data of an *n*-of-1 trial is to visualize the data without doing any statistical analysis at all. When the number of repeated measures within the individual patient is relatively high, it is possible to use time series analysis. With this method, the development over time in a particular outcome is analyzed taking into account the correlation of the repeated measures within the patient. This correlation is known as the autocorrelation. One of the advantages of using time series analysis is to build forecast models. With these models the unobserved development over time in an outcome variable for a particular patient can be predicted from the observed development over time and the magnitude of the autocorrelation. Furthermore, several covariates can be added to the time series analysis in order to investigate the influence of these covariates on the development and on the forecast. The detailed description of the use of time series analysis in *n*-of-1 trials and forecast models go beyond the scope of this book. For more information one is referred to McCleary and Hay (1980), Box and Jenkins (1994), Wei (2013), and Peixeiro (2019). Although, they have some potential, it should be realized that time series analysis and forecast models are not much used in the analysis of *n*-of-1 trials.

J. W. R. Twisk, *Analysis of Data from Randomized Controlled Trials*, https://doi.org/10.1007/978-3-030-81865-4_7

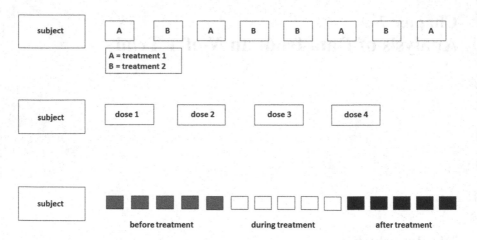

Fig. 7.1   Illustration of different *n*-of-1 trials

It should further be realized that a classical *n*-of-1 trial design is not much used in practice. Although many authors claim to perform such a study, in real life, most of the studies are multiple *n*-of-1 trials performed in multiple patients. These series of *n*-of-1 trials are basically not really *n*-of-1 trials. In fact these studies are comparable to a regular RCT with only a few patients. Why these studies are often mentioned *n*-of-1 trials is because in many situations the intervention or treatment under study is developed for the individual patient.

7.2   Example

A nice example of a series of *n*-of-1 trials is a study performed by de Raaij et al. (unpublished data). In this study a few patients, who received a highly personalized physiotherapy treatment were followed for a period of time.

The example dataset includes a series of 7 *n*-of-1 trials. The seven patients received a personalized physiotherapy treatment in order to decrease pain intensity. There were on average 6 measurements (either 5 or 6) for each patient before treatment, on average 7 measurements (ranging between 5 and 10) during treatment, and on average 11 measurements (ranging between 8 and 13) after treatment. The goal of the analysis was to estimate the effect of the personalized physiotherapy treatment. Table 7.1 shows the descriptive information regarding pain intensity at the three periods for the seven patients.

From Table 7.1 it can be seen that for most patients the personalized treatment is highly effective to reduce pain, although for patient 4, there is no decrease in pain both in the treatment period as well as in the after treatment period. Furthermore, it can be seen that for some of the patients (patient 1 and 3), the personalized intervention reduces pain only in the treatment period, while for other patients

Table 7.1 Mean and standard deviation (between brackets) of pain intensity for the seven patients at the three periods

	Before treatment	During treatment	After treatment
Pain intensity:			
Patient 1	7.5 (1.4)	3.4 (1.8)	4.2 (1.5)
Patient 2	6.8 (1.9)	4.1 (2.1)	1.8 (2.2)
Patient 3	3.8 (1.3)	1.2 (1.1)	1.4 (1.4)
Patient 4	7.7 (0.8)	7.7 (0.8)	8.2 (0.6)
Patient 5	8.5 (0.5)	5.2 (3.0)	1.5 (0.5)
Patient 6	6.2 (0.4)	4.8 (1.5)	1.5 (1.2)
Patient 7	2.3 (0.5)	1.3 (0.8)	0.7 (0.6)

Table 7.2 Data structure needed to analyze a series of N-of-1 trials

Id	Outcome	Period	Time
1	Y_{t1}	1	1
1	Y_{t2}	1	2
1	Y_{t3}	1	3
.	.	.	.
1	Y_{t6}	2	6
1	Y_{t7}	2	7
1	Y_{t8}	2	8
.	.	.	.
1	Y_{t11}	3	11
1	Y_{t12}	3	12
1	Y_{t13}	3	13

(patient 2, 5, 6, and 7), the decrease in the treatment period is followed by a decrease in the after treatment period as well. Besides this, it is also clear that the before treatment pain level is highly different between the patients.

Although just the description of the data provides a lot of information, when a series of 1-of-n trials is performed, it also possible to analyze the data with a mixed model analysis in order to estimate the treatment effect including a 95% confidence interval and corresponding p-value. A mixed model analysis is of course necessary to take into account the dependency of the observations within the patient. In this mixed model analysis, in the present example, the period (i.e., before treatment, during treatment, and after treatment) is used as independent variable, because the aim of the analysis was to investigate the difference in average pain between the three periods (Eq. 7.1):

$$Y_t = \beta_0 + \beta_1 \times period_1 + \beta_2 \times period_2 \tag{7.1}$$

where Y_t = outcome measured at the different measurements, $period_1$ = dummy variable for period 1, β_1 = overall intervention effect in period 1; $period_2$ = dummy variable for period 2, and β_2 = overall intervention effect in period 2.

```
Mixed-effects ML regression                     Number of obs      =       169
Group variable: patient                         Number of groups   =         7

                                                Obs per group:
                                                          min =         22
                                                          avg =       24.1
                                                          max =         27

                                                Wald chi2(2)       =    103.58
Log likelihood = -340.82253                     Prob > chi2        =    0.0000

-------------------------------------------------------------------------------
       pain |      Coef.   Std. Err.      z    P>|z|     [95% Conf. Interval]
------------+------------------------------------------------------------------
     period |
     during |  -2.050147    .359916    -5.70   0.000    -2.755569   -1.344725
      after |  -3.312681   .3257602   -10.17   0.000    -3.951159   -2.674202
            |
      _cons |    6.09317   .7808287     7.80   0.000     4.562774    7.623566
-------------------------------------------------------------------------------


-------------------------------------------------------------------------------
  Random-effects Parameters  |   Estimate   Std. Err.     [95% Conf. Interval]
-----------------------------+-------------------------------------------------
Patient: Identity            |
                var(_cons)   |   3.779058   2.083825      1.282388    11.13648
-----------------------------+-------------------------------------------------
               var(Residual) |    2.86033   .3178153      2.300584    3.556267
-------------------------------------------------------------------------------
LR test vs. linear model: chibar2(01) = 117.35       Prob >= chibar2 = 0.0000
```

Output 7.1 Results of the mixed model analysis to obtain an overall treatment effect in the series of *n*-of-1 trials

Table 7.2 shows the structure of the data used to estimate the parameters for the example dataset.

In the analysis, the before treatment period was used as reference category. Output 7.1 shows the result of this analysis.

Like all other mixed model analyses, Output 7.1 contains three parts. In the upper part, it can be seen that seven patients are included in the analysis. In total 169 observations were made, and it can be seen that on average there were 24.1 observations per patient. In the second part of the output (i.e., the fixed part of the model), the regression coefficients for the two dummy variables for the during treatment period and the after treatment period are given. The regression coefficient for the dummy variable for the during treatment period (-2.050147) indicates the difference in average pain between the during treatment period and the before treatment period. The regression coefficient for the dummy variable for the after treatment period (-3.312681) indicates the difference in average pain between the after treatment period and the before treatment period. For both differences also the 95% confidence intervals are given and the corresponding *p*-values, which show that both differences are highly significant. From the last part of the output (the random part of the model), it can be seen that the variance in pain between the patients is relatively high compared to the residual variance. In Sect. 4.2 it was already explained that the two variances can be used to calculate the intraclass correlation coefficient (ICC). The ICC can be calculated by dividing the between patient variance (3.799) by the total variance (3.799 + 2.860). In the present example, the ICC equals 57%.

```
Mixed-effects ML regression                    Number of obs     =        169
Group variable: patient                        Number of groups  =          7

                                               Obs per group:
                                                            min =         22
                                                            avg =       24.1
                                                            max =         27

                                               Wald chi2(2)      =     103.58
Log likelihood = -340.82253                    Prob > chi2       =     0.0000

-------------------------------------------------------------------------------
       pain |      Coef.   Std. Err.      z    P>|z|     [95% Conf. Interval]
------------+------------------------------------------------------------------
     period |
     before |    2.050147    .359916    5.70   0.000     1.344725    2.755569
      after |   -1.262534   .3108614   -4.06   0.000    -1.871811   -.6532566
            |
      _cons |    4.043023    .774153    5.22   0.000     2.525711    5.560335
-------------------------------------------------------------------------------


-------------------------------------------------------------------------------
  Random-effects Parameters |   Estimate   Std. Err.     [95% Conf. Interval]
----------------------------+--------------------------------------------------
patient: Identity           |
                 var(_cons) |   3.779058   2.083825      1.282388    11.13648
----------------------------+--------------------------------------------------
              var(Residual) |    2.86033   .3178153      2.300584    3.556267
-------------------------------------------------------------------------------
LR test vs. linear model: chibar2(01) = 117.35        Prob >= chibar2 = 0.0000
```

Output 7.2 Results of the mixed model analysis to obtain an overall treatment effect in the series of n-of-1 trials with the during treatment period as reference category

To obtain the average pain difference between the after treatment period and the during treatment period, the two regression coefficients for the two dummy variables reported in Output 7.1 can be subtracted from each other. In this case this difference is equal to -3.312681 minus $-2.050147 = -1.262534$. To obtain the 95% confidence interval around this difference and the corresponding p-value, the same analysis can be redone, with the during treatment period (or the after treatment period) as reference category. Output 7.2 shows the result of the analysis with the during treatment period as reference category.

In Output 7.2 it can be seen that indeed the difference in average pain between the after treatment period and the during treatment period equals -1.262534. The 95% confidence interval ranges between -1.871811 and -0.6532566, and the corresponding p-value is <0.001.

The results reported in Outputs 7.1 and 7.2 are based on a series of 1-of-n trials and report the overall effect of the personalized treatment. However, in Table 7.1 it could be seen that the treatment response is quite different for some of the patients. So, the next step in the analysis is trying to find characteristics of the patients with a certain treatment response. One of the possibilities is to add interaction terms with the particular characteristics to the model. In the example dataset, for instance, anxiety is measured during the study. Anxiety is measured as a time-dependent continuous variable (i.e., at all repeated measures anxiety is measured) on a scale from 1 to 10. Output 7.3 shows the result of the analysis including the interaction with anxiety.

```
Mixed-effects ML regression                  Number of obs      =        169
Group variable: patient                      Number of groups   =          7

                                             Obs per group:
                                                          min =         22
                                                          avg =       24.1
                                                          max =         27

                                             Wald chi2(5)       =     186.11
Log likelihood = -318.15545                  Prob > chi2        =     0.0000


---------------------------------------------------------------------------------
        pain |     Coef.    Std. Err.      z     P>|z|    [95% Conf. Interval]
-------------+-------------------------------------------------------------------
      period |
      during |  -2.955427    .5047852   -5.85    0.000   -3.944788   -1.966066
       after |   -3.53871    .4315614   -8.20    0.000   -4.384555   -2.692865
             |
     anxiety |   .2371204    .1009303    2.35    0.019    .0393007    .4349402
             |
     period#|
   c.anxiety |
      during |   .4353413    .1476739    2.95    0.003    .1459058    .7247769
       after |   .5336566    .1629122    3.28    0.001    .2143547    .8529586
             |
       _cons |   5.385839    .6096682    8.83    0.000    4.190911    6.580767
---------------------------------------------------------------------------------


---------------------------------------------------------------------------------
  Random-effects Parameters  |   Estimate   Std. Err.     [95% Conf. Interval]
-----------------------------+---------------------------------------------------
patient: Identity            |
                var(_cons)  |   1.600728    .9419898     .5051336    5.072582
-----------------------------+---------------------------------------------------
              var(Residual) |   2.241414    .249485     1.802093    2.787832
---------------------------------------------------------------------------------
LR test vs. linear model: chibar2(01) = 45.91        Prob >= chibar2 = 0.0000
```

Output 7.3 Results of the mixed model analysis to obtain an overall treatment effect in the series of *n*-of-1 trials including the interaction with anxiety

The most important result from Output 7.3 can be found in the fixed part of the model, i.e., the interaction between period and anxiety. It can be seen that both interaction terms are statistically significant ($p = 0.003$ and $p = 0.001$, respectively) and both regression coefficients are positive (0.4353413 and 0.5336566, respectively). The positive regression coefficients indicate that the higher the anxiety score of the patient, the less effective the individualized treatment is. The regression coefficients themselves indicate that for a one unit higher anxiety, the difference in average pain between the during treatment period and the before treatment period is 0.4353413 less big, while the difference between the after treatment period and the before treatment period is 0.5336566 less big. Based on these results, it is not surprising that patient 4 has the highest average anxiety score in the dataset (see Table 7.3).

Assuming that not many patients are included in a series of *n*-of-1 trials, it should be realized that the reliability of results obtained from the analysis of a series of *n*-of-1 trials highly depends on the number of repeated measurements within the patient. When there are only a few repeated measurements for each patient, adding interaction terms to the mixed model analysis, for instance, will be hardly possible due to a lack of power.

Table 7.3 Mean and standard deviation (between brackets) of anxiety for the seven patients at the three periods

Pain intensity	Before treatment	During treatment	After treatment
Patient 1	2.8 (3.1)	1.0 (0.0)	1.1 (0.3)
Patient 2	1.2 (2.7)	3.7 (2.8)	1.5 (0 0.8)
Patient 3	0.2 (0.4)	0.0 (0.0)	0.0 (0.0)
Patient 4	4.3 (0.5)	4.0 (0.0)	4.6 (0.8)
Patient 5	5.8 (1.3)	2.2 (1.3)	1.2 (0.4)
Patient 6	4.5 (2.1)	3.5 (1.8)	0.0 (0.0)
Patient 7	1.5 (0.8)	1.3 (0.5)	0.1 (0.3)

Although the use of n-of-1 trials has gained popularity in the last decade, in the literature not much information is available regarding the analysis of data from n-of-1 trials. However, some further reading can, for instance, be found in Lillie et al. (2011) and Chen and Chen (2014).

Chapter 8
Dichotomous Outcomes

8.1 Introduction

In the foregoing chapters, all examples had a continuous outcome variable. It is, of course also possible that the outcome variable in an RCT is not continuous. The theory behind the analysis of RCT data with other outcomes is comparable to what has been discussed for continuous outcomes. Only a different regression method must be used. When, for instance, the outcome variable in an RCT is dichotomous, logistic regression has to be used to estimate treatment effects. When there is only one follow-up measurement, regular logistic regression analysis can be used, while in an RCT with more than one follow-up measurement, longitudinal logistic regression analysis can be used. With dichotomous outcomes, mostly an adjustment for baseline differences in the outcome between the intervention group and the control group is not necessary, because at baseline mostly all subjects are either scoring 1 or 0 (depending on the coding of the particular outcome variable). Suppose that the aim of an RCT is to estimate the effect of a new treatment against hypertension; in the (source) population all subjects must have hypertension. In other words, they all have the same value of the outcome at baseline. When this is not the case, i.e., when there is a difference in the baseline dichotomous outcome between the intervention and the control group, the situation is slightly more complicated than described for continuous outcomes. This has to do with a phenomenon which is called non-collapsibility (see Sect. 8.5).

8.2   RCT with a Dichotomous Outcome with One Follow-Up Measurement

To illustrate the analysis of RCT data with a dichotomous outcome variable and only one follow-up measurement, an example dataset is derived from an RCT aimed to assess the effectiveness of a classification-based treatment approach compared to usual physiotherapy care in patients with subacute or chronic low back pain (Apeldoorn et al., 2012). The outcome variable of interest was functional status, which was measured with the ten-item Oswestry Disability Index (ODI), with higher scores indicating lower functional status. The maximum score on the ODI is 50, and in the present study, a cutoff value of 12 was used to distinguish between good (<12) and bad (≥12) functional status. The outcome variable was assessed 52 weeks after the start of treatment. Table 8.1 shows descriptive information, and Output 8.1 shows the results of the logistic regression analysis to estimate the intervention effect. It should be noted that in this example bad functional status is coded 1 and that all patients in the RCT had a bad functional status at baseline.

The output of the logistic regression analysis contains two parts. The first part shows some general information including the number of observations (140), the log likelihood, and the overall p-value for the model. The second part contains the regression coefficients from which the regression coefficient for the group variable (−0.5362828) is of course the most interesting. The coefficient indicates the difference in the outcome at week 52 between the intervention and control groups. The problem with logistic regression is that the outcome is not easy to interpret. The outcome is the natural log of the odds to have a bad functional status. Because of this difficult interpretation, the regression coefficient obtained from a logistic regression analysis is mostly transformed into an odds ratio. The odds ratio can be calculated by taking the e-power of the regression coefficient. Output 8.2 shows the result of the

Table 8.1   Descriptive information (number and percentage of subjects) regarding the functional status trial

	Good functional status	Bad functional status
Intervention group	46 (68.7%)	21 (31.3%)
Control group	41 (56.2%)	32 (43.8%)

```
Logistic regression                          Number of obs    =        140
                                             LR chi2(1)       =       2.33
                                             Prob > chi2      =     0.1269
Log likelihood = -91.705466                  Pseudo R2        =     0.0125

------------------------------------------------------------------------------
     status |      Coef.   Std. Err.      z    P>|z|     [95% Conf. Interval]
------------+-----------------------------------------------------------------
      group |  -.5362828   .3535512    -1.52   0.129    -1.22923     .1566647
      _cons |  -.2478362   .2358818    -1.05   0.293    -.7101561    .2144838
------------------------------------------------------------------------------
```

Output 8.1   Results of a logistic regression analysis in order to obtain an intervention effect in the functional status trial

```
Logistic regression                          Number of obs    =      140
                                             LR chi2(1)       =     2.33
                                             Prob > chi2      =   0.1269
Log likelihood = -91.705466                  Pseudo R2        =   0.0125


-----------------------------------------------------------------------------
   status | Odds Ratio   Std. Err.      z     P>|z|     [95% Conf. Interval]
----------+------------------------------------------------------------------
    group |  .5849185    .2067986     -1.52   0.129     .2925176    1.169603
    _cons |  .7804878    .1841029     -1.05   0.293     .4915675    1.239222
-----------------------------------------------------------------------------
```

Output 8.2 Results of a logistic regression analysis in order to obtain an intervention effect in the functional status trial showing the odds ratio

```
   Source |       SS           df       MS       Number of obs   =      140
----------+------------------------------------   F(1, 138)       =     2.32
    Model |  .545201098         1  .545201098     Prob > F        =   0.1298
 Residual |  32.3905132       138  .234713864     R-squared       =   0.0166
----------+------------------------------------   Adj R-squared   =   0.0094
    Total |  32.9357143       139  .236947585     Root MSE        =   .48447


-----------------------------------------------------------------------------
   status |    Coef.    Std. Err.      t     P>|t|      [95% Conf. Interval]
----------+------------------------------------------------------------------
    group | -.1249233    .0819662     -1.52   0.130    -.2869953    .0371486
    _cons |  .4383562    .0567032      7.73   0.000     .3262366    .5504757
-----------------------------------------------------------------------------
```

Output 8.3 Results of a linear regression analysis in order to obtain the risk difference in the functional status trial

logistic regression analysis to obtain the effect of the intervention showing the odds ratio instead of the regression coefficient.

From Output 8.2 it can be seen that the odds ratio equals 0.5849185. This means that the odds for having a bad functional status in the intervention group is 0.58 times as high as the odds for having a bad functional status in the control group. The 95% confidence interval around this odds ratio ranges from 0.2925176 to 1.169603, and the corresponding p-value equals 0.129.

It is sometimes argued that an odds ratio is not the best effect estimate to report when an RCT is performed with a dichotomous outcome. This has to do with the fact that an RCT is a prospective study and that, therefore, better a risk difference or relative risk can be reported. The risk difference can be easily obtained by performing a linear regression analysis with the dichotomous outcome. This method is highly controversial because the assumptions of a linear regression analysis do not hold for dichotomous outcomes. The outcome is not continuous and is totally not normally distributed. However, when a linear regression analysis is performed with the dichotomous outcome, the regression coefficient nicely indicates the risk difference (see Output 8.3).

The regression coefficient for the group variable (−0.1249233) indicates the difference in the outcome (the dichotomous variable good functional status versus bad functional status) between the intervention and control groups, which is basically the risk difference between the two groups. Linear regression analysis can be used for dichotomous outcomes, but because of its controversial use, this chapter will continue with logistic regression analysis for the dichotomous outcomes and, therefore, with odds ratios as effect estimates.

8.3   RCT with a Dichotomous Outcome with More Than One Follow-Up Measurement

It has already been mentioned (see Chap. 3) that the two most frequently used regression-based methods to analyze data from an RCT with more than one follow-up measurement are mixed model analysis and generalized estimating equations (GEE analysis). In Chap. 3, it was explained that the general idea of both methods is that an adjustment is made for the dependency of the repeated observations within the subject. In mixed model analysis, this adjustment is performed by modeling the difference between the subjects (i.e., the between-subject variance) (Goldstein, 2003; Laird & Ware, 1982), while in GEE analysis this adjustment is performed by modeling directly the within-subject correlation (Liang & Zeger, 1986; Zeger & Liang, 1986). Because the correlation within the subject is essentially the same as the difference between the subjects, the estimated regression coefficients may be expected to be the same in both methods. It was mentioned that the only difference between the two methods was the way missing data was handled. Because mixed model analysis is slightly better than GEE analysis in dealing with missing data, all analyses of RCT data with a continuous outcome and more than one follow-up measurement were performed with linear mixed model analyses.

However, there is also another difference between the two methods. GEE analysis is known as a population average approach, while mixed model analysis is known as a subject-specific approach (Twisk, 2013; Twisk et al., 2017). This does not influence the values of the estimated regression coefficients obtained from a linear GEE analysis and a linear mixed model analysis, but it does influence the values of the estimated regression coefficients obtained from a logistic GEE analysis and a logistic mixed model analysis. The difference in regression coefficients is a theoretical one, which is always in favor of a mixed model analysis, meaning that the regression coefficients obtained from a logistic mixed model analysis will always be "higher" (i.e., further away from zero) compared to the regression coefficients obtained from a logistic GEE analysis. This difference is based on a mathematical relationship and depends on the magnitude of the between-subject variance (see Eq. 8.1a, Eq. 8.1b) (Heo & Leon, 2005; ten Have et al., 2004). When there is more between-subject variance, the difference between the regression coefficients will be larger:

$$\beta^{(pa)} = \left[\left(\frac{16\sqrt{3}}{15\pi} \right)^2 \sigma_b^2 \right]^{-1/2} \beta^{(ss)} \tag{8.1a}$$

$$\frac{16\sqrt{3}}{15\pi} = 0.588 \tag{8.1b}$$

where $\beta^{(pa)}$ = population average regression coefficient obtained from a logistic GEE analysis, σ_b^2 = between-subject variance, and $\beta^{(ss)}$ = subject-specific regression coefficient obtained from a logistic mixed model analysis.

Both GEE analysis and mixed model analysis are used for the analysis of longitudinal data with a dichotomous outcome variable, but from the literature it is not clear which of the two methods should be used and which regression coefficients should be reported (Heo & Leon, 2005; Hu et al., 1998; Hubbard et al., 2010). As for continuous outcomes, it is sometimes argued that mixed model analysis should be preferred above GEE analysis because mixed model analysis is more suitable to deal with missing data (Albert, 1999; Omar et al., 1999; Twisk, 2013). However, in the next sections, it will be shown that it is the other way round, i.e., it is better to use a logistic GEE analysis to obtain effect estimates in an RCT with a dichotomous outcome variable and more than one follow-up measurement.

8.3.1   Example

The example dataset is derived from a three-arm RCT regarding an Internet-based treatment for adults with depressive symptoms (Warmerdam et al., 2008). Besides a waiting list (WL) group, two interventions were evaluated, i.e., an Internet-based problem-solving therapy (PST) and an Internet-based cognitive behavioral therapy (CBT). As outcome variable, self-reported depression (measured with the Center for Epidemiological Studies Depression scale (CES-D)) was measured at 5, 8, and 12 weeks. The CES-D is widely used for identifying subjects with depression, and a score of 16 or higher is considered to represent clinical depression (Table 8.2).

Because at baseline all subjects suffered from clinical depression, an adjustment for the baseline value is not necessary. Therefore, a longitudinal logistic regression analysis can be performed to estimate the treatment effects (see Eq. 8.2):

$$ln\left(odds(Y_t = 1)\right) = \beta_0 + \beta_1 X_1 + \beta_2 X_2 \tag{8.2}$$

where Y_t = dichotomous outcome measured at the three follow-up measurements, X_1 = dummy variable for treatment variable 1, X_2 = dummy variable for treatment

Table 8.2 The number and percentage (between brackets) of subjects with clinical depression for the three groups at the three follow-up measurements regarding the Internet RCT

	5 weeks	8 weeks	12 weeks
Waiting list	60 (84.5%)	54 (76.1%)	52 (82.5%)
Problem-solving therapy	47 (77.1%)	28 (54.9%)	26 (56.2%)
Cognitive behavioral therapy	30 (57.7%)	30 (58.8%)	23 (54.8%)

```
Mixed-effects logistic regression              Number of obs      =        508
Group variable:                   id           Number of groups   =        205

                                               Obs per group:
                                                             min =          1
                                                             avg =        2.5
                                                             max =          3

Integration method: mvaghermite                Integration pts.   =          7

                                               Wald chi2(2)       =      12.34
Log likelihood = -275.23898                    Prob > chi2        =     0.0021
-----------------------------------------------------------------------------
    clindep |      Coef.    Std. Err.      z    P>|z|     [95% Conf. Interval]
------------+----------------------------------------------------------------
intervention |
        PST |  -1.415105    .5170469    -2.74   0.006    -2.428498   -.4017113
        CBT |  -1.753144    .5313925    -3.30   0.001    -2.794655   -.7116343
            |
      _cons |   2.447067    .4226946     5.79   0.000     1.618601    3.275533
------------+----------------------------------------------------------------
id          |
  var(_cons)|   4.714806    1.524432                      2.501763    8.885495
-----------------------------------------------------------------------------
LR test vs. logistic model: chibar2(01) = 53.60          Prob >= chibar2 = 0.0000
```

Output 8.4 Results of the logistic mixed model analysis to estimate the overall intervention effect on average over time in the Internet RCT (PST = problem-solving therapy, CBT = cognitive behavioral therapy)

variable 2, β_1 = overall treatment effect for X_1, and β_2 = overall treatment effect for X_2.

The first analysis is an analysis to estimate the overall treatment effect on average over time. Because the results of the logistic mixed model analysis are different from the logistic GEE analysis, both results will be reported. Output 8.4 shows the results of the logistic mixed model analysis, while Output 8.5 shows the results of the logistic GEE analysis.

The output of a logistic mixed model analysis is similar to the output of a linear mixed model analysis. It also includes three parts. The first part gives some general information of the model and the data used for the analysis. It can be seen that a logistic mixed model analysis is performed and that the cluster variable is the subject (id). This indicates that an adjustment is made for the correlated (repeated) observations within the subject. Furthermore, it can be seen that 508 observations are made within 205 subjects and that the average number of observations within a patient is 2.5. The output also shows the log likelihood and the integration method (mvaghermite). The latter stands for mean-variance adaptive Gauss-Hermite quadrature, which is the relatively complicated mathematical method to calculate the log likelihood in a logistic mixed model analysis. A detailed explanation about this method goes beyond the scope of this book; see for mathematical details, for instance, Liu and Pierce (1994), Lesaffre and Spiessens (2001), or Rabe-Hesketh and Skrondal (2001). The second part of the output (the fixed part of the model) shows the regression coefficients. The coefficient for PST indicates the difference in the outcome on average over time between the group who received problem-solving therapy and the waiting list group. The coefficient for CBT indicates the difference in the outcome on average over time between the group who received cognitive

```
Mixed-effects logistic regression              Number of obs       =        508
Group variable:                 id             Number of groups    =        205

                                               Obs per group:
                                                            min =          1
                                                            avg =        2.5
                                                            max =          3

Integration method: mvaghermite                Integration pts.    =          7

                                               Wald chi2(2)        =      12.34
Log likelihood = -275.23898                    Prob > chi2         =     0.0021
------------------------------------------------------------------------------
    clindep |     exp(b)   Std. Err.      z    P>|z|     [95% Conf. Interval]
------------+-----------------------------------------------------------------
intervention |
        PST |   .2429002   .1255908    -2.74   0.006     .0881692     .6691739
        CBT |   .1732284   .0920523    -3.30   0.001     .061136      .4908414
            |
      _cons |   11.55441   4.883986     5.79   0.000     5.046025     26.45733
------------+-----------------------------------------------------------------
id          |
   var(_cons)|   4.714806   1.524432                     2.501763     8.885495
------------------------------------------------------------------------------
LR test vs. logistic model: chibar2(01) = 53.60        Prob >= chibar2 = 0.0000
```

Output 8.5 Results of the logistic mixed model analysis to estimate the overall intervention effect on average over time in the Internet RCT reporting odds ratios (PST = problem-solving therapy, CBT = cognitive behavioral therapy)

behavioral therapy and the waiting list group. As has been mentioned before, the outcome in a logistic model is the natural log of the odds of being clinically depressed. Because of the complicated interpretation, the regression coefficients are transformed into odds ratios, which are normally reported as effect estimates. Output 8.5 shows the same results as has been shown in Output 8.4 but now reporting odds ratios.

From the fixed part in Output 8.5, it can be seen that the odds ratio for problem-solving therapy versus waiting list is 0.2429002, which indicates that the odds of being clinically depressed on average over time for the subjects in the problem-solving therapy group is 0.24 times as high as the odds of being clinically depressed for the subjects in the waiting list group. For cognitive behavioral therapy versus waiting list, the odds ratio is 0.1732284. The output also gives the 95% confidence intervals around the odds ratios and the corresponding p-values.

The last part of the outputs (Outputs 8.4 and 8.5) contain the random part of the model. The random part of a logistic mixed model analysis only contains the random intercept variance (4.714806) which indicates the difference in the outcome between the subjects. The output does not give a residual variance. This is different from the output of linear mixed model analysis and due to the fact that a logistic regression model does not have a residual variance. Basically the model estimates the probability of having the outcome (i.e., clinical depression) and that probability is estimated without error. In fact, the error is outside the model when the probability is compared to the observed value. The observed value is either zero (for no clinical depression) or one (for yes clinical depression), while the probability is a value somewhere between zero and one.

```
GEE population-averaged model                      Number of obs      =        508
Group variable:                           id       Number of groups   =        205
Link:                                  logit       Obs per group:
Family:                             binomial                   min =          1
Correlation:                     exchangeable                   avg =        2.5
                                                                max =          3
                                                   Wald chi2(2)       =      12.09
Scale parameter:                          1        Prob > chi2        =     0.0024

                                   (Std. Err. adjusted for clustering on id)
-------------------------------------------------------------------------------
             |             Robust
    clindep  |     Coef.   Std. Err.      z    P>|z|     [95% Conf. Interval]
-------------+-----------------------------------------------------------------
intervention |
         PST |  -.8435477    .308191    -2.74   0.006    -1.447591   -.2395044
         CBT | -1.062383    .3227646    -3.29   0.001     -1.69499   -.4297759
             |
       _cons |  1.442273    .2329943     6.19   0.000     .9856124    1.898933
-------------------------------------------------------------------------------
```

Output 8.6 Results of the logistic GEE analysis to estimate the overall intervention effect on average over time in the Internet RCT (PST = problem-solving therapy, CBT = cognitive behavioral therapy)

The same analysis can also be performed with a logistic GEE analysis. As has been mentioned before, GEE analysis adjusts for the correlated observations within the subject by assuming a certain correlation structure (see Sect. 3.4). For logistic GEE analysis, mostly an exchangeable correlation structure is chosen. Firstly because this structure is the most efficient due to the fact that only one parameter has to be estimated and, secondly, because logistic GEE analysis is quite robust against a wrong choice for the correlation structure (Twisk, 2013). Output 8.6 shows the result of the logistic GEE analysis.

The output of a logistic GEE analysis is similar to the output of a linear GEE analysis (see Chap. 3). The only difference is the link function and the family. The logit link and the binomial family indicate that a logistic regression analysis is performed. In Chap. 3 (see Output 3.4), it was seen that a linear regression analysis was indicated by an identity link and a Gaussian family. Furthermore, the scale parameter which was an indication of the unexplained variance in the output of the linear GEE analysis is now set to 1. This is because, as has been mentioned before, there is no residual variance in the logistic model. The regression coefficients shown in the second part of the output have exactly the same interpretation as the ones obtained from a logistic mixed model analysis. The regression coefficient for problem-solving therapy (−0.8435477) indicates the difference in the outcome on average over time between the group who received problem-solving therapy and the waiting list group. The coefficient for cognitive behavioral therapy (−1.062383) indicates the difference in the outcome on average over time between the group who received cognitive behavioral therapy and the waiting list group. Also here, the outcome is the natural log of the odds of being clinically depressed, and, again, because of the complicated interpretation, the regression coefficients are transformed into odds ratios, which are normally reported as effect estimates. Output 8.7 shows the same results as has been shown in Output 8.6 but now reporting odds ratios.

```
GEE population-averaged model                    Number of obs      =      508
Group variable:                            id    Number of groups   =      205
Link:                                   logit    Obs per group:
Family:                              binomial                  min  =        1
Correlation:                     exchangeable                  avg  =      2.5
                                                               max  =        3
                                                 Wald chi2(2)       =    12.09
Scale parameter:                            1    Prob > chi2        =   0.0024

                                        (Std. Err. adjusted for clustering on id)
--------------------------------------------------------------------------------
             |              Robust
    clindep  | Odds Ratio  Std. Err.      z    P>|z|     [95% Conf. Interval]
-------------+------------------------------------------------------------------
intervention |
        PST  |  .4301817   .1325781    -2.74   0.006      .235136    .7870178
        CBT  |  .3456312   .1115575    -3.29   0.001     .1836011    .6506549
             |
       _cons |  4.230299   .9856354     6.19   0.000     2.679452    6.678765
--------------------------------------------------------------------------------
```

Output 8.7 Results of the logistic GEE analysis to estimate the overall intervention effect on average over time in the Internet RCT reporting odds ratios (PST = problem-solving therapy, CBT = cognitive behavioral therapy)

From Output 8.7 it can be seen that the odds ratio for problem-solving therapy versus waiting list is 0.4301817, and for cognitive behavioral therapy versus waiting list the odds ratio is 0.3456312. The interpretation of the odds ratios is (of course) exactly the same as the interpretation of the odds ratios provided by the logistic mixed model analysis. Again, the output also gives the 95% confidence interval around the odds ratios and the corresponding p-values.

As expected, the regression coefficients and therefore also the odds ratios show stronger effects when they are estimated with the logistic mixed model analysis than with the logistic GEE analysis.

The next step in the analysis is to estimate the effect of the interventions at the different follow-up measurements. To obtain those effect estimates, time (represented with two dummy variables) and the interaction between the intervention variables and time were added to the model (Eq. 8.3):

$$
\begin{aligned}
ln\left(odds(Y_t = 1)\right) = {} & \beta_0 + \beta_1 X_1 + \beta_2 X_2 + \beta_3 time_2 + \beta_4 time_3 + \beta_5 X_1 \\
& \times time_2 + \beta_6 X_1 \times time_3 + \beta_7 X_2 \times time_2 + \beta_8 X_2 \\
& \times time_3
\end{aligned}
\tag{8.3}
$$

where Y_t = dichotomous outcome measured at the three follow-up measurements; X_1 = dummy variable for treatment variable 1; X_2 = dummy variable for treatment variable 2; β_1 = treatment effect for X_1, at the first follow-up measurement; β_2 = treatment effect for X_2 at the first follow-up measurement; and $time_2$ and $time_3$ = dummy variables for the second and third follow-up measurement.

Output 8.8 shows the result of the logistic mixed model analysis with the first follow-up measurement as reference category.

The odds ratios for the two intervention conditions reported in Output 8.8 are the odds ratios estimated at the first follow-up measurement. So, the odds ratio for

```
Mixed-effects logistic regression          Number of obs     =      508
Group variable:                id          Number of groups  =      205

                                           Obs per group:
                                                       min =        1
                                                       avg =      2.5
                                                       max =        3

Integration method: mvaghermite            Integration pts.  =        7

                                           Wald chi2(8)      =    23.29
Log likelihood = -266.46199                Prob > chi2       =   0.0030
--------------------------------------------------------------------------
    clindep |    exp(b)    Std. Err.      z    P>|z|    [95% Conf. Interval]
------------+-------------------------------------------------------------
            |
intervention|
        PST |   .4249087    .321936    -1.13   0.259    .0962442   1.875929
        CBT |   .0925714   .0718584    -3.07   0.002    .0202178   .4238586
            |
       time |
          2 |   .3841377   .2229583    -1.65   0.099    .1231513   1.198215
          3 |   .5538669   .3434857    -0.95   0.341    .1642574   1.867609
            |
intervention#|
       time |
      PST#2 |   .3602031   .2993099    -1.23   0.219    .0706714    1.83591
      PST#3 |   .2620149   .2288382    -1.53   0.125    .0473048   1.451266
      CBT#2 |   2.552884   2.069003     1.16   0.248    .5213976   12.49952
      CBT#3 |   1.621419   1.395443     0.56   0.574    .3001405   8.759226
            |
       _cons|   24.49095   15.53652     5.04   0.000    7.063531   84.91596
------------+-------------------------------------------------------------
id          |
  var(_cons)|   6.217744   2.077234                     3.230443   11.96751
--------------------------------------------------------------------------
LR test vs. logistic model: chibar2(01) = 61.53       Prob >= chibar2 = 0.0000
```

Output 8.8 Results of the logistic mixed model analysis including an interaction between intervention and time in the Internet RCT reporting odds ratios (PST = problem-solving therapy, CBT = cognitive behavioral therapy)

problem-solving therapy compared to waiting list equals 0.4249087, while the odds ratio for cognitive behavioral therapy compared to waiting list equals 0.0925714. To obtain the odds ratios for both interventions compared to waiting list at the other two follow-up measurements, the same analysis has to be done with a different reference category for time. Output 8.9 and Output 8.10 show the output of these analyses.

The same three analyses can also be performed with a logistic GEE analysis. Outputs 8.11, 8.12, and 8.13 show the results of these analyses.

To illustrate the differences between the results obtained from the logistic mixed model analyses and the logistic GEE analyses, Table 8.3 summarizes the results.

From Table 8.3 it is obvious that all odds ratios obtained from the logistic mixed model analyses provide stronger effects than the ones obtained from the logistic GEE analysis. The question then arises, which of the two results should be reported? To answer that question, for all logistic models, the predicted probabilities were calculated (see Eq. 8.4):

```
Mixed-effects logistic regression              Number of obs      =        508
Group variable:                    id          Number of groups   =        205

                                               Obs per group:
                                                          min =          1
                                                          avg =        2.5
                                                          max =          3
Integration method: mvaghermite                Integration pts.   =          7

                                               Wald chi2(8)        =      23.29
Log likelihood = -266.46199                    Prob > chi2         =     0.0030
-------------------------------------------------------------------------------
   clindep |    exp(b)   Std. Err.      z     P>|z|     [95% Conf. Interval]
-----------+-------------------------------------------------------------------
intervention |
       PST |   .1530534   .1112796   -2.58   0.010     .03681      .6363863
       CBT |   .2363242   .1710586   -1.99   0.046     .0571983    .9764131
           |
      time |
         1 |   2.603233   1.510949    1.65   0.099     .8345745    8.120092
         3 |   1.441845   .8261522    0.64   0.523     .4690235    4.432435
           |
intervention#|
      time |
     PST#1 |   2.776211   2.306886    1.23   0.219     .544689     14.15
     PST#3 |   .7274089   .5886132   -0.39   0.694     .1489338    3.552743
     CBT#1 |   .3917138   .3174671   -1.16   0.248     .0800031    1.917922
     CBT#3 |   .635132    .5257142   -0.55   0.583     .1254018    3.216801
           |
      _cons |   9.407897   5.104916    4.13   0.000     3.247979    27.25033
-----------+-------------------------------------------------------------------
id         |
var(_cons) |   6.217744   2.077234                     3.230443    11.96751
-------------------------------------------------------------------------------
LR test vs. logistic model: chibar2(01) = 61.53      Prob >= chibar2 = 0.0000
```

Output 8.9 Results of the logistic mixed model analysis including the interaction between intervention and time with the second follow-up measurement as reference time point in the Internet RCT reporting odds ratios (PST = problem-solving therapy, CBT = cognitive behavioral therapy)

$$P(y = 1) = 1/1 + e^{-\beta_0 + \beta_1 X_1 + \dots} \qquad (8.4)$$

where $P(y = 1)$ = predicted probability and $\beta_0 + \beta_1 X_1 + \dots$ = logistic regression model.

The predicted probabilities obtained from the different analyses can then be compared to the observed percentages shown in Table 8.2. Table 8.4 shows the predicted probabilities of having clinical depression at the different follow-up measurements.

Figure 8.1 shows the predicted probabilities from the two analyses and the observed percentages for the three groups at the three follow-up measurements.

Figure 8.1 shows clearly that the predicted probabilities based on the regression coefficients of the logistic GEE analyses are much closer to the observed percentages than the predicted probabilities based on the regression coefficients of the logistic mixed model analyses. This indicates that the effect estimates obtained from the logistic mixed model analyses are overestimations of the "real" effects. The difference between the observed percentages and the predicted probabilities by the logistic GEE analyses are caused by the missing observations in the dataset. When the same comparison would have been made in a dataset without missing data, the observed

```
Mixed-effects logistic regression          Number of obs      =         508
Group variable:              id            Number of groups   =         205

                                           Obs per group:
                                                       min =           1
                                                       avg =         2.5
                                                       max =           3

Integration method: mvaghermite            Integration pts.   =           7

                                           Wald chi2(8)       =       23.29
Log likelihood = -266.46199                Prob > chi2        =      0.0030
------------------------------------------------------------------------------
   clindep |     exp(b)   Std. Err.       z    P>|z|    [95% Conf. Interval]
-----------+------------------------------------------------------------------
intervention |
       PST |    .1113324   .0866056    -2.82   0.005    .0242366    .5114131
       CBT |    .1500971   .1171346    -2.43   0.015    .0325163    .6928564
           |
      time |
         1 |    1.805488   1.11969      0.95   0.341    .5354439    6.088006
         2 |    .693556    .3973957    -0.64   0.523    .2256096    2.132089
           |
intervention#|
      time |
     PST#1 |    3.816576   3.333315     1.53   0.125    .6890536    21.13951
     PST#2 |    1.374743   1.11243      0.39   0.694    .2814726    6.714391
     CBT#1 |    .6167439   .530789     -0.56   0.574    .1141653    3.331773
     CBT#2 |    1.574476   1.303232     0.55   0.583    .3108678    7.974368
           |
      _cons |   13.56473   7.951404     4.45   0.000    4.299834    42.79277
-----------+------------------------------------------------------------------
id         |
  var(_cons)|  6.217744   2.077234                     3.230443    11.96751
------------------------------------------------------------------------------
LR test vs. logistic model: chibar2(01) = 61.53      Prob >= chibar2 = 0.0000
```

Output 8.10 Results of the logistic mixed model analysis including the interaction between intervention and time with the third follow-up measurement as reference time point in the Internet RCT reporting odds ratios (PST = problem-solving therapy, CBT = cognitive behavioral therapy)

percentages would have been exactly the same as the predicted probabilities obtained from the logistic GEE analyses (Twisk et al., 2017). Therefore, it is strongly advised to use logistic GEE analysis instead of logistic mixed model analysis to obtain effect estimates in RCTs with dichotomous outcome variables and with more than one follow-up measurement.

8.4   Comments

There are several papers in which a logistic GEE analysis (a population average approach) is compared to a logistic mixed model analysis (a subject-specific approach). Most of these comparisons were made on cross-sectional data with clustering of data on, for instance, neighborhood level, school level, etc. Although the directions of the differences were comparable to the ones observed in the Internet RCT example, the magnitude of the differences were, in general, much lower (Bellamy et al., 2009; Kim et al., 2006). This is due to the fact that the between-cluster differences in these cross-sectional studies were much lower than the

```
GEE population-averaged model                      Number of obs      =       508
Group variable:                          id        Number of groups   =       205
Link:                                 logit        Obs per group:
Family:                            binomial                         min =         1
Correlation:                   exchangeable                         avg =       2.5
                                                                    max =         3
                                                   Wald chi2(8)       =     25.06
Scale parameter:                          1        Prob > chi2        =    0.0015

                                          (Std. Err. adjusted for clustering on id)
------------------------------------------------------------------------------
                |               Robust
    clindep     | Odds Ratio  Std. Err.      z    P>|z|    [95% Conf. Interval]
----------------+-------------------------------------------------------------
intervention    |
          PST   |  .6176652   .2849051    -1.04   0.296    .2501075   1.525385
          CBT   |  .2592947   .1137991    -3.08   0.002    .1097031    .6128701
                |
         time   |
            2   |  .5728581   .1719119    -1.86   0.063    .3181308   1.031546
            3   |  .7114194   .2910829    -0.83   0.405    .3190435   1.586359
                |
intervention#   |
         time   |
        PST#2   |  .5785234    .279993    -1.13   0.258    .2240565   1.493772
        PST#3   |  .4856061   .2656687    -1.32   0.187    .1661892   1.418944
        CBT#2   | 1.735226    .7216842     1.33   0.185    .7679612   3.920781
        CBT#3   | 1.314181    .7077188     0.51   0.612    .4573643   3.776141
                |
        _cons   | 5.772432   1.947254      5.20   0.000    2.980006   11.18151
------------------------------------------------------------------------------
```

Output 8.11 Results of the logistic GEE analysis including the interaction between intervention and time in the Internet RCT reporting odds ratios (PST = problem-solving therapy, CBT = cognitive behavioral therapy)

between-cluster (subject) differences within a longitudinal study. It was already mentioned that the magnitude of the differences between the results of the two methods depend on the magnitude of the between-cluster/between-subject variance (see Eq. 8.1). Surprisingly, in none of the papers comparing logistic GEE analysis with logistic mixed model analysis, a recommendation is provided which of the two methods should be used. It is sometimes argued that preferring one method above the other depends on the research question to be answered (Hu et al., 1998; Subramanian, 2004). In general, if one is interested in the regression coefficient, i.e., the effect estimate, a population average approach should be used, and when one is interested in estimating the heterogeneity between subjects in a longitudinal study or between clusters in a cross-sectional study, a subject-specific approach should be used. In RCTs, one is not interested in the heterogeneity between subjects, but one is interested in the effect estimates, taking into account the dependency of the observations within the subjects. For this purpose, logistic GEE analysis provides a valid estimate of the coefficient, while logistic mixed model analysis does not.

```
GEE population-averaged model                    Number of obs      =        508
Group variable:                             id   Number of groups   =        205
Link:                                    logit   Obs per group:
Family:                               binomial                      min =         1
Correlation:                      exchangeable                      avg =       2.5
                                                                    max =         3
                                                 Wald chi2(8)       =      25.06
Scale parameter:                             1   Prob > chi2        =     0.0015

                                          (Std. Err. adjusted for clustering on id)
-------------------------------------------------------------------------------
             |             Robust
     clindep | Odds Ratio  Std. Err.      z    P>|z|     [95% Conf. Interval]
-------------+-----------------------------------------------------------------
intervention |
         PST |  .3573338   .1417012   -2.60   0.009     .1642589    .7773545
         CBT |  .4499347   .1780122   -2.02   0.044     .2071954    .9770548
             |
        time |
           1 |  1.745633   .5238557    1.86   0.063     .9694191    3.143361
           3 |  1.241877   .4098609    0.66   0.512     .6503597    2.371393
             |
intervention#|
        time |
       PST#1 |  1.728538   .8365756    1.13   0.258     .6694462    4.463159
       PST#3 |  .8393888   .3635414   -0.40   0.686     .3591746    1.961646
       CBT#1 |   .576294    .239682   -1.33   0.185     .2550512    1.302149
       CBT#3 |  .7573547   .3415324   -0.62   0.538     .3129293    1.832957
             |
       _cons |  3.306785   .9255162    4.27   0.000     1.910593    5.723262
-------------------------------------------------------------------------------
```

Output 8.12 Results of the logistic GEE analysis including the interaction between intervention and time with the second follow-up measurement as reference time point in the Internet RCT reporting odds ratios (PST = problem-solving therapy, CBT = cognitive behavioral therapy)

8.4.1 Missing Data

One of the arguments against the use of a logistic GEE analysis is that the results of a logistic GEE analysis are biased when there is missing data, especially when the missing data is not completely at random (Little, 1995; Twisk, 2013). In most longitudinal RCTs, there is missing data, and in most longitudinal RCTs, the missing data is not completely at random. So, it is a common belief that a logistic GEE analysis should not be used in those situations. Although this argument is theoretically true, it should be realized that the percentage of missing data must be very high to have a detrimental influence on the validity of the results of a (logistic) GEE analysis (Twisk, 2013). In the analyses performed on the example dataset, it is not clear what the impact of the missing data is on the estimation of the intervention effect(s). However, looking at the predicted probabilities from both the logistic GEE analyses and the logistic mixed model analyses, the influence of missing data is probably not very big. In all analyses the comparison between the predicted probabilities and the observed percentages was in favor of the logistic GEE analyses. This is despite the fact that the missing data in the example dataset was not completely at random and that the percentage of missing data was around 17% which is relatively high for an RCT.

```
GEE population-averaged model                        Number of obs     =        508
Group variable:                              id      Number of groups  =        205
Link:                                     logit      Obs per group:
Family:                                binomial                    min =          1
Correlation:                       exchangeable                    avg =        2.5
                                                                   max =          3
                                                     Wald chi2(8)      =      25.06
Scale parameter:                             1       Prob > chi2       =     0.0015

                                          (Std. Err. adjusted for clustering on id)
-------------------------------------------------------------------------------
                |             Robust
      clindep   | Odds Ratio  Std. Err.     z    P>|z|     [95% Conf. Interval]
----------------+--------------------------------------------------------------
intervention    |
          PST   |   .299942   .1270838   -2.84   0.004    .1307338    .6881557
          CBT   |  .3407602   .1483046   -2.47   0.013    .1452083    .7996614
                |
         time   |
            1   |  1.405641    .575129    0.83   0.405    .6303742    3.134369
            2   |  .8052327   .2657537   -0.66   0.512     .421693    1.537611
                |
intervention#   |
         time   |
        PST#1   |  2.059282   1.126606    1.32   0.187    .7047493    6.017236
        PST#2   |  1.191343   .5159737    0.40   0.686    .5097759    2.784161
        CBT#1   |  .7609301   .4097796   -0.51   0.612    .2648206    2.186441
        CBT#2   |  1.320385   .5954336    0.62   0.538    .5455664     3.19561
                |
        _cons   |   4.10662    1.27683    4.54   0.000    2.232693    7.553358
-------------------------------------------------------------------------------
```

Output 8.13 Results of the logistic GEE analysis including the interaction between intervention and time with the third follow-up measurement as reference time point in the Internet RCT reporting odds ratios (PST = problem-solving therapy, CBT = cognitive behavioral therapy)

Table 8.3 Summary of the odds ratios and 95% confidence intervals (between brackets) obtained from the logistic mixed model analyses and the logistic GEE analyses to obtain treatment effects in the Internet RCT

	Logistic mixed model analysis	Logistic GEE analysis
Overall on average over time		
PST	0.24 (0.09 to 0.67)	0.43 (0.24 to 0.79)
CBT	0.17 (0.06 to 0.49)	0.35 (0.18 to 0.65)
First follow-up		
PST	0.42 (0.10 to 1.88)	0.62 (0.25 to 1.53)
CBT	0.09 (0.02 to 0.42)	0.26 (0.11 to 0.61)
Second follow-up		
PST	0.15 (0.04 to 0.64)	0.36 (0.16 to 0.78)
CBT	0.24 (0.06 to 0.98)	0.45 (0.25 to 0.98)
Third follow-up		
PST	0.11 (0.02 to 0.51)	0.30 (0.13 to 0.69)
CBT	0.15 (0.03 to 0.69)	0.34 (0.15 to 0.80)

PST = problem-solving therapy, CBT = cognitive behavioral therapy

Table 8.4 Predicted probabilities of having clinical
depression from the logistic
mixed model analysis and the
logistic GEE analysis regarding the Internet RCT

	Waiting list	PST	CBT
First follow-up			
Logistic mixed model	96%	91%	69%
Logistic GEE analysis	85%	78%	60%
Second follow-up			
Logistic mixed model	90%	59%	69%
Logistic GEE analysis	77%	54%	60%
Third follow-up			
Logistic mixed model	93%	60%	67%
Logistic GEE analysis	80%	55%	58%

PST = problem-solving therapy, CBT = cognitive behavioral
therapy

8.4.2   Hypothesis Testing Versus Effect Estimation

It is sometimes argued that logistic GEE analysis and logistic mixed model analysis
can be used interchangeably, because both the regression coefficients and the
standard errors are "higher" (i.e., further away from zero) in a more or less
systematical manner when they are derived from a logistic mixed model analysis
compared to a logistic GEE analysis. Consequently, the p-values and the answer to
the question whether there is a significant difference between the intervention(s) and
the control group are similar between the two statistical methods. When one is only
interested in hypothesis testing, this is a valid argument, but nowadays, the major
interest of analyzing data from an RCT is the magnitude of the effect estimate rather
than hypothesis testing. And because the effect estimates are highly different
between the two methods, it is important to make the right choice.

8.4.3   Cluster RCT with a Dichotomous Outcome

In Chap. 4, the analysis of data from a cluster RCT was discussed. It was mentioned
that mixed model analysis can be used to take into account the correlated observations within the cluster. When a cluster RCT has a dichotomous outcome, the same
problems with the use of mixed model analysis occur as has been mentioned earlier
in this chapter. However, when there is only one follow-up measurement, the
differences between the results obtained from a logistic GEE analysis and a logistic
mixed model analysis will be less pronounced. This is because the between-cluster
variance is much lower than the between-subject variance obtained in an RCT with
more than one follow-up measurement. Therefore, the difference between the
regression coefficients will be relatively small (see Eq. 8.1). When a cluster RCT
is performed with more than one follow-up measurement, besides the correlated
observations of the repeated measurements within the subject, there are also correlated observations within the cluster, i.e., the data has a three-level structure. When

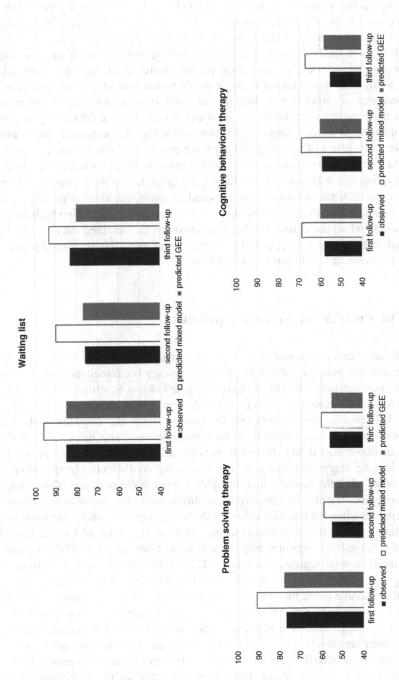

Fig. 8.1 Predicted probabilities of having clinical depression from the logistic mixed model analysis and the logistic GEE analysis regarding the Internet RCT and observed percentages of patients with clinical depression

the number of clusters is relatively large, i.e., when an adjustment for the cluster variable by adding dummy variables to the model is not possible, a logistic GEE analysis cannot be used anymore because within a (logistic) GEE analysis, it is not possible to take into account clustering on more than one level. In Chap. 4 it was shown that mixed model analysis is capable of dealing with clustering on more than one level, so when also the correlation on the cluster level must be taken into account, a (logistic) mixed model analysis should be used with the same "problems" as has been shown earlier in this chapter. The simplest solution to this "problem" is to ignore the correlation on the cluster level and to use a logistic GEE analysis only taking into account the correlated observations of the repeated measurements within the subject. The effect of ignoring this approach depends, of course, on the magnitude of the between-cluster variance. When the between-cluster variance is relatively small, ignoring this variance will not have a big influence on the estimation of the regression coefficients and corresponding standard errors. An alternative solution is to use a logistic mixed model analysis taking into account the correlation both on the subject level and on the cluster level and to transform the obtained subject-specific regression coefficients into population average regression coefficients by using Eq. 8.1. However, this solution is not much used in practice.

8.5   The Problem of Non-Collapsibility

It has already been mentioned that in an RCT with a dichotomous outcome, an adjustment for the baseline value is mostly not necessary because in most RCTs with a dichotomous outcome, all subjects have the same value at baseline (see Sect. 8.1). When this is not the case, i.e., when there is a difference in the baseline dichotomous outcome between the intervention and the control group, the situation is slightly more complicated than described for continuous outcomes. This has to do with the problem of non-collapsibility. Non-collapsibility deals with the fact that in (longitudinal) logistic regression analysis, the regression coefficients change when a variable is added to the model which is highly related to the outcome. This change in regression coefficient is irrespective of the difference in this variable between the two groups. So when the baseline values of the two groups are exactly the same and the baseline value is (highly) related to the outcome, the result of the unadjusted (longitudinal) logistic regression analysis will differ from the result of the adjusted (longitudinal) logistic regression analysis. This is different from a (longitudinal) linear regression analysis. When the groups at baseline are exactly the same, adding the baseline variable to the linear model will not influence the regression coefficient, even when the particular variable is highly related to the outcome. That was also the reason why an adjustment for time did not make sense in an RCT with more than one follow-up measurement (see Sect. 3.7). It was mentioned that time was not related to the intervention variable (i.e., the intervention and control groups are measured at the same time points), and, therefore, time could not influence the magnitude of the regression coefficients. Theoretically, this non-collapsibility phenomenon arises from differences in the total variances between a logistic regression analysis with and a logistic regression analysis without the adjustment for the particular variable. In a linear model, the total variance is the summation of explained and unexplained variance. When a covariate is added to a linear regression model, the unexplained variance decreases, while the explained variance increases with the same amount. However, in a logistic model, the unexplained variance is a fixed number. So when a covariate that is related to the outcome is added to a logistic model which only contains the intervention variable, the total variance will increase. Because of this increased variance, it is often said that, adding a variable to the logistic model that is related to the outcome changes the scale on which the regression coefficients must be interpreted (Greenland & Robins, 2009; Hernan et al., 2011; Newman, 2004).

8.5.1 A Numerical Example

The non-collapsibility phenomenon, which is not known by most researchers, is illustrated with the numerical example shown in Table 8.5.

The numerical example includes 240 subjects equally divided into an intervention group and a control group. In this illustration, it can be seen that there is no difference in baseline values between the intervention and control groups. For both groups half of the subjects have 0, and half of the subjects have 1 at baseline. Because in the intervention group, 100 subjects have 1, and 20 subjects have 0 at the follow-up measurement, while in the control group, half of the subjects have 1 and half of the subjects have 0 at the follow-up measurement, the crude intervention effect (i.e., without adjusting for the baseline value) gives an odds ratio of 5. It can further be seen that the baseline value is highly related to the outcome variable. For the subjects with a baseline value of 1, 100 subjects have 1, and 20 subjects have 0 at the follow-up measurement. For the subjects with a baseline value of 0, half of the subjects have 0 and half of the subjects have 1 at the follow-up measurement. The corresponding odds ratio, therefore, also equals 5. Because the baseline value is exactly the same for both the intervention and control groups, an adjustment for the baseline value should not change the estimation of the treatment effect. However,

Table 8.5 Dataset used to illustrate the problem of non-collapsibility

Intervention	Outcome at baseline	Outcome at follow-up	Number of subjects
0	0	0	45
0	0	1	15
0	1	0	15
0	1	1	45
1	0	0	15
1	0	1	45
1	1	0	5
1	1	1	55

```
Logistic regression                              Number of obs    =      240
                                                 LR chi2(2)       =    67.07
                                                 Prob > chi2      =   0.0000
Log likelihood = -119.22613                      Pseudo R2        =   0.2195

------------------------------------------------------------------------------
     outcome | Odds Ratio   Std. Err.      z    P>|z|     [95% Conf. Interval]
-------------+----------------------------------------------------------------
intervention |   6.694644    2.296889    5.54   0.000     3.417321    13.11503
    baseline |   6.694644    2.296889    5.54   0.000     3.417321    13.11503
       _cons |   .3864882    .102894    -3.57   0.000     .2293626    .6512534
------------------------------------------------------------------------------
```

Output 8.14 Result of the logistic regression analysis based on the data of the numerical example adjusted for baseline

when a logistic regression analysis is performed adjusting for the baseline value, the adjusted odds ratio is around 6.7, which is much higher than the expected odds ratio of 5 (see Output 8.14).

In the situation described in the numerical example, there is no difference in the outcome variable at baseline between the intervention group and the control group. If this situation is observed in a real-life RCT, an adjustment for the baseline value is not necessary and will, therefore, not be applied and the effect estimates will be valid. However, when there is a difference in the baseline value of the outcome between the two groups, an adjustment for the baseline differences will be applied to take into account regression to the mean. The adjusted effect estimate can then be biased by this non-collapsibility phenomenon. In this situation, the change in regression coefficient which occurs when the baseline value is added to the model is partly caused by regression to the mean and partly by non-collapsibility. So, in that case the results of the logistic regression analysis adjusted for the baseline should be interpreted with great caution.

However, although the non-collapsibility phenomenon can lead to biased effect estimates, it should be realized that in most RCTs with a dichotomous outcome all subjects will have the same value at baseline. So, in most RCTs with a dichotomous outcome, an adjustment for the baseline value will not be necessary.

8.6   Other Outcomes

It is of course also possible that the outcome variable of an RCT is not continuous or dichotomous. In the beginning of this chapter it was already mentioned that the theory behind the analysis of RCT data with other outcomes is comparable to what has been discussed for continuous outcomes. Only a different regression method must be used. When, for instance, the outcome variable in an RCT is a count (e.g., the number of complaints, the number of injuries, etc.), Poisson regression analysis can be used to estimate treatment effects, and when there is more than one follow-up measurement, Poisson mixed model analysis can be used. When the outcome variable in an RCT has a floor or ceiling effect, Tobit regression analysis can be used to estimate treatment effects, and when there is more than one follow-up measurement, Tobit mixed model analysis can be used. When the outcome variable in an RCT is a survival outcome (i.e., a dichotomous event and the time to that event), Cox regression can be used to estimate treatment effects, etc. Although it should be noted that when the outcome variable is a survival outcome, there is only one outcome for each subject. Because of that, in the analysis an adjustment for the correlated observations within the subject is not necessary. It is beyond the scope of this book to discuss all the analyses of RCT data with different outcomes in great detail, but it is important to realize that all the principles discussed in this book also hold for the analysis of RCT data with other outcomes.

Chapter 9
What to Do When Only a Baseline Measurement Is Available

9.1 Introduction

In Chaps. 2 and 3, it has been discussed that in the analyses of RCT data, it is recommended to use an analysis of covariance in which the follow-up measurement (s) are used as the outcome, whereas the baseline value is used as a covariate. Therefore, a problem arises when a baseline measurement is available for a particular subject, while all follow-up measurements are missing. The intention-to-treat principle states that these subjects should be analyzed according to their assigned condition (see Sect. 1.2). Yet, in an analysis adjusted for the baseline value, the data of these subjects cannot be included in the analysis. There is a lot of discussion going on about how to deal with these subjects. Some researchers argue that data of these subjects should not be taken into account in the analysis, as no data is available on the follow-up measurements after treatment initiation. Others argue that not including data of these subjects in the analysis drives against the principle of intention-to-treat and leads to bias in the effect estimates. In other words, how to deal with subjects with only a baseline value in the analysis of RCT data remains unclear (Gravel et al., 2007; Hollis & Campbell, 1999; Mukaka et al., 2016; White et al., 2012; Wright & Sim, 2003).

Several suggestions are provided in the literature on analyzing RCT data to deal with the above mentioned problem. The most classical solution is to impute the follow-up measurement(s) with the baseline value carried forward (European Medicines Agency, 2010). Although highly criticized, this method is still widely used. Multiple imputations using more complicated imputation methods (such as predictive mean matching) are suggested as a better alternative (Morris et al., 2014; van Buuren, 2007). The advantage of predictive mean matching, when compared to other multiple imputation methods, is that it imputes values that are observed in the dataset and are therefore much alike real values. And although it is not an issue in this chapter, this makes the method suitable for normally distributed outcome variables as well as non-normally distributed outcome variables. The general idea behind predictive mean matching is that first predictive values are generated for all subjects (including the subjects with no missing data). Secondly, based on the predictive values, a group of subjects without missing data (in the examples of this chapter a group of five subjects is used) is selected that are close to the predictive values of a subject with missing data. From this group of subjects, one subject is randomly selected, and the observed value of this particular subject is used for the imputation. This procedure is then repeated several times to create multiple imputed datasets.

In Chap. 3 it was discussed that when there is more than one follow-up measurement available, a mixed model analysis can be performed to estimate treatment effects. In such as mixed model analysis, data of subjects with a baseline measurement but missing follow-up measurements are mostly ignored (i.e., are not part of the analysis). This is based on the idea that the use of a mixed model analysis (adjusting for the baseline value) is enough to deal with the missing data. However, although it is true that a mixed model analysis is suitable for the analysis of longitudinal data with outcome missingness, the subjects with only a baseline value are not included in the analysis, because no follow-up outcome measurements are available. To deal with this phenomenon, the alternative repeated measures analysis can be used (see Sect. 3.4.2). In this alternative repeated measures analysis the baseline value is part of the longitudinal outcome, and the model is estimated without the inclusion of the intervention variable but with time and the interaction between intervention and time. Due to the fact that the intervention variable is not part of the model, the intercept of such an analysis reflects the combined baseline value for both the intervention and control groups. In this alternative repeated measures analysis, the regression coefficient for the interaction between intervention and time indicates the treatment effect (see Sect. 3.4.2).

Because there remains heterogeneity in applied methods to deal with the problem of missing data on all follow-up measurements while the baseline value is available, the purpose of this chapter is to illustrate the different methods used to deal this problem.

9.2   Examples

9.2.1   RCT with One Follow-Up Measurement

The example is taken from an intervention study in which the effectiveness of a long-term homocysteine-lowering treatment with folic acid plus pyridoxine in reducing systolic blood pressure was evaluated (van Dijk et al., 2001). In this example a baseline measurement and one follow-up measurement were performed. Table 9.1 shows the descriptive information regarding the baseline values for the patients with and without follow-up measurements.

From Table 9.1 it can be seen that around 6% of the patients only had a baseline measurement and that the patients with only a baseline measurement have a much

Table 9.1 Mean and standard deviation (between brackets) of the baseline systolic blood pressure

	Baseline systolic blood pressure (mmHg)
Subjects with follow-up ($N = 130$)	128.4 (15.4)
Subjects with only baseline ($N = 9$)	132.2 (15.1)

```
Mixed-effects ML regression              Number of obs     =        130

                                         Wald chi2(2)      =     133.09
Log likelihood = -490.07319              Prob > chi2       =     0.0000

------------------------------------------------------------------------
  systolic |     Coef.   Std. Err.      z    P>|z|    [95% Conf. Interval]
-----------+------------------------------------------------------------
  sys_base |    .654648   .0606359   10.80   0.000    .5358039    .7734922
 treatment |  -4.379276   1.864113   -2.35   0.019   -8.032871   -.7256818
     _cons |   44.49622   8.028237    5.54   0.000    28.76117    60.23128
------------------------------------------------------------------------


------------------------------------------------------------------------
  Random-effects Parameters  |   Estimate   Std. Err.    [95% Conf. Interval]
-----------------------------+------------------------------------------
                var(Residual)|   110.1354   13.66061      86.36711   140.4447
------------------------------------------------------------------------
```

Output 9.1 Results of the analysis of covariance on the complete cases to estimate the treatment effect

higher baseline systolic blood pressure compared to the patients for whom a follow-up measurement is available. As has been mentioned before, there are several methods available to estimate the effect of the treatment in this particular situation. The mostly used method is to perform an analysis of covariance on the complete cases, i.e., the 130 patients with both a baseline measurement and a follow-up measurement. Output 9.1 shows the result of this analysis of covariance.

From Output 9.1 it can be seen that the analysis is performed on 130 patients. The effect estimate (i.e., the regression coefficient) for the treatment variable (-4.379276) indicates the difference in systolic blood pressure between the treatment group and the control group at the follow-up measurement, adjusted for the baseline value of systolic blood pressure. Note that the analysis is performed within a mixed model framework. This is of course not necessary, because there is only one systolic blood pressure for each patient used as outcome. However, the results are the same as the results from a regular linear regression analysis.

The reason for using the mixed model framework is that the second possibility to estimate the treatment effect uses both the baseline and the follow-up measurement as outcome. As has been mentioned before, this method is known as the alternative repeated measures analysis (see Sects. 3.4.2 and 9.1). The advantage of this method is that all patients are included in the analysis. Due to the fact that both the baseline and the follow-up measurement for each patient are used as outcome, the analysis has to be performed with a mixed model analysis to take into account the correlated observations within the patient. Output 9.2 shows the result of this analysis.

From the first part of Output 9.2, it can be seen that all 139 patients are used in the analysis. In the second part of the output, the fixed part of the model, it can be seen

```
Mixed-effects ML regression                  Number of obs     =        269
Group variable: patient                      Number of groups  =        139

                                             Obs per group:
                                                          min =          1
                                                          avg =        1.9
                                                          max =          2

                                             Wald chi2(2)      =       8.90
Log likelihood = -1067.0493                  Prob > chi2       =     0.0117

-------------------------------------------------------------------------------
    systolic |      Coef.   Std. Err.      z    P>|z|     [95% Conf. Interval]
-------------+-----------------------------------------------------------------
        time |  -.0070504   1.377082    -0.01   0.996    -2.706081     2.69198
 int_time_t~r |  -4.206756   1.896396    -2.22   0.027    -7.923624   -.4898875
       _cons |   128.6475   1.267921   101.46   0.000     126.1624    131.1326
-------------------------------------------------------------------------------


-------------------------------------------------------------------------------
  Random-effects Parameters  |   Estimate   Std. Err.     [95% Conf. Interval]
-----------------------------+-------------------------------------------------
id: Identity                 |
                  var(_cons) |   154.4051   23.40379      114.7207    207.8172
-----------------------------+-------------------------------------------------
                var(Residual)|   69.05465   8.584891      54.12169    88.10783
-------------------------------------------------------------------------------
LR test vs. linear model: chibar2(01) = 82.94         Prob >= chibar2 = 0.0000
```

Output 9.2   Result of the alternative repeated measures analysis to estimate the treatment effect

that the adjustment for the baseline value is performed by adding time and the interaction between treatment and time to the model. The estimated intercept (128.6475) indicates the overall baseline value averaged over the treatment and control group. Because the same baseline value is estimated for the two groups, the effect estimate is adjusted for the observed differences at baseline between the two groups. The effect estimate is given by the regression coefficient for the interaction between treatment and time (−4.206756). The interpretation is, of course, the same as the interpretation of the effect estimate derived from the analysis of covariance (see Output 9.1). Output 9.2 also contains a random part with a random intercept variance. As has been mentioned before, adding a random intercept on patient level to the model is necessary to adjust for the dependent observations within the patient.

Besides the analysis of covariance on the complete cases or the alternative repeated measures analysis, it is also possible to impute the missing follow-up data. The classical way to impute the missing follow-up data is a single imputation based on the last value carried forward. With this method, the baseline value is carried forward to the follow-up measurement. The general idea of this method is that there is no change over time. After the last values carried forward imputation, an analysis of covariance is performed to estimate the treatment effect. Output 9.3 shows the result of this analysis.

The difference between the analysis of covariance performed on the complete cases and the analysis of covariance performed on the last value carried forward imputed dataset is the fact that the latter is performed on 139 patients instead of 130 patients. The estimated treatment effect is again given by the regression

```
Mixed-effects ML regression                  Number of obs    =        139

                                             Wald chi2(2)     =     155.27
Log likelihood = -521.09886                  Prob > chi2      =     0.0000

------------------------------------------------------------------------------
    systolic |      Coef.   Std. Err.      z    P>|z|     [95% Conf. Interval]
-------------+----------------------------------------------------------------
systolic_b~e |   .6809099   .0574194    11.86   0.000     .5683699    .7934499
      therap |  -3.849872   1.760067    -2.19   0.029    -7.299541   -.4002036
       _cons |    41.0918   7.601838     5.41   0.000     26.19247    55.99113
------------------------------------------------------------------------------


------------------------------------------------------------------------------
  Random-effects Parameters  |   Estimate   Std. Err.     [95% Conf. Interval]
-----------------------------+------------------------------------------------
                var(Residual)|   105.6306   12.67061          83.5    133.6267
------------------------------------------------------------------------------
```

Output 9.3 Results of the analysis of covariance on the last value carried forward imputed dataset to estimate the treatment effect

coefficient for the treatment variable. In the last value carried forward imputed dataset, the treatment effect is equal to -3.849872.

Slightly more sophisticated is the use of multiple imputation. In this example predictive mean matching is used for the multiple imputation (see Sect. 9.1), and the imputation model included the baseline value of the outcome and the treatment variable. Although the rule of thumb is that the number of imputations is more or less equal to the percentage of missing data, in this example 20 imputed datasets were generated. Also in this situation an analysis of covariance is performed to estimate the treatment effect. To obtain one effect estimate after the multiple imputation, first an analysis of covariance is performed on the 20 imputed datasets. Then, the average value of the 20 effect estimates is calculated. This average value is known as the pooled effect estimate. Slightly more complicated is the estimation of the pooled standard error of the effect estimate. This pooled standard error contains two components. The first component is the average of the standard errors of the 20 analyses performed. The second component is based on the differences between the effect estimates obtained from the 20 analyses. This second component indicates the uncertainty of the imputations. Output 9.4 shows the result of the pooled analysis of covariance performed on the multiple imputed datasets.

The first part of Output 9.4 shows some general information of the dataset used and the imputations. It can, for instance, be seen that 20 imputations were performed and that the analysis is performed on 139 subjects. Because the focus of this book is not on imputation methods, the general information regarding the imputation will not be discussed in detail. More interesting is the part of the output that contains the pooled regression coefficients. The regression coefficient for the treatment variable (-4.143669) indicates the effect estimate. The interpretation is of course exactly the same as the effect estimates derived from the other methods.

Table 9.2 gives an overview of the results derived from the four analyses performed.

From Table 9.2 it can be seen that the alternative repeated measures analysis and the multiple imputation provided more or less the same effect estimate. The complete

```
Multiple-imputation estimates                   Imputations      =          20
Mixed-effects ML regression                     Number of obs    =         139
                                                Average RVI      =      0.0926
                                                Largest FMI      =      0.1113
DF adjustment:     Large sample                 DF:     min      =    1,565.19
                                                        avg      =    2,333.51
                                                        max      =    3,261.52
Model F test:      Equal FMI                    F(  2, 3987.7)   =       64.12
                                                Prob > F         =      0.0000


--------------------------------------------------------------------------------
   systolic_ |     Coef.    Std. Err.       t    P>|t|     [95% Conf. Interval]
-------------+------------------------------------------------------------------
 systolic_b~e |  .6636646    .0615467    10.78   0.000      .5429905    .7843387
   treatment |  -4.143669   1.922132     -2.16   0.031     -7.913894   -.3734443
       _cons |  43.32352    8.171624      5.30   0.000      27.30063    59.3464
--------------------------------------------------------------------------------


--------------------------------------------------------------------------------
 Random-effects Parameters  |   Estimate   Std. Err.    [95% Conf. Interval]
----------------------------+---------------------------------------------------
              var(Residual) |  112.01005   14.39522       87.32116   143.67953
--------------------------------------------------------------------------------
```

Output 9.4 Results of the analysis of covariance on the multiple imputed datasets to estimate the treatment effect

Table 9.2 Overview of the results derived from the different methods

	Effect Estimate	95% CI	p-value
Complete case analysis	−4.38	−8.03 to −0.73	0.019
Alternative repeated measures	−4.21	−7.92 to −0.49	0.027
Last value carried forward	−3.85	−7.30 to −0.40	0.029
Multiple imputation	−4.14	−7.91 to −0.37	0.031

case analysis provided a slightly higher effect estimate, while the last value carried forward imputation provided a slightly lower effect estimate.

9.2.2   RCT with More Than One Follow-Up Measurement

The second example dataset is derived from a three-arm RCT regarding an Internet-based treatment for adults with depressive symptoms (Warmerdam et al., 2008). Besides a waiting list (WL) group, two interventions were evaluated, i.e., an Internet-based problem-solving therapy (PST) and an Internet-based cognitive behavioral therapy (CBT). The same example was also used in Chap. 8, where the analysis of an RCT with a dichotomous outcome was discussed. In the present example self-reported depression (measured with the Center for Epidemiological Studies Depression scale (CES-D)) was used as continuous outcome. Depression was measured at baseline and after 5, 8, and 12 weeks. Table 9.3 shows the descriptive information regarding the baseline values for the subjects with and without follow-up measurements.

Table 9.3 Mean and standard deviation (between brackets) of baseline depression

	Baseline depression
Subjects with at least one follow-up ($N = 205$)	31.3 (7.4)
Subjects with only baseline ($N = 58$)	33.0 (7.9)

```
Mixed-effects ML regression              Number of obs     =        508
Group variable: id                       Number of groups  =        205

                                         Obs per group:
                                                      min  =          1
                                                      avg  =        2.5
                                                      max  =          3

                                         Wald chi2(3)      =      69.00
Log likelihood = -1764.5387              Prob > chi2       =     0.0000

------------------------------------------------------------------------------
  depression |    Coef.   Std. Err.     z    P>|z|    [95% Conf. Interval]
-------------+----------------------------------------------------------------
intervention |
         PST | -4.528607  1.429431   -3.17   0.002   -7.330241   -1.726974
         CBT | -5.209772  1.46398    -3.56   0.000   -8.07912    -2.340424
             |
  dep_basel~e |  .5766133  .0818199    7.05   0.000    .4162493    .7369773
        _cons |  7.112022  2.777835    2.56   0.010   1.667565    12.55648
------------------------------------------------------------------------------


------------------------------------------------------------------------------
  Random-effects Parameters  |   Estimate   Std. Err.    [95% Conf. Interval]
-----------------------------+------------------------------------------------
id: Identity                 |
                 var(_cons)  |   59.14884    7.33685     46.38343     75.4275
-----------------------------+------------------------------------------------
               var(Residual) |   30.47558    2.481812    25.97966    35.74954
------------------------------------------------------------------------------
LR test vs. linear model: chibar2(01) = 188.50      Prob >= chibar2 = 0.0000
```

Output 9.5 Results of the longitudinal analysis of covariance on the non-imputed dataset to estimate the overall intervention effect on average over time in the Internet RCT (PST = problem-solving therapy, CBT = cognitive behavioral therapy)

From Table 9.3 it can be seen that in this example around 22% of the subjects only had a baseline value and that baseline depression was slightly higher for the subjects with only a baseline value compared to the subjects with at least one follow-up measurement.

Basically, for an RCT with more than one follow-up measurement, the same methods can be used to deal with the problem of availability of a baseline value but missing follow-up measurement. So, the first analysis that is performed is a longitudinal analysis of covariance on the available data. One must realize that this analysis is not a complete case analysis, because subjects only need one follow-up measurement to be included in the analysis. The reason why this is possible has to do with the fact that using a mixed model analysis is one of the recommended methods to deal with missing outcomes in a longitudinal study (Twisk et al., 2013). When there is more than one follow-up measurement, the data to be analyzed is longitudinal, so therefore, all subjects with at least one follow-up measurement are part of the analysis. Output 9.5 shows the result of the longitudinal analysis of covariance.

```
Mixed-effects ML regression                    Number of obs      =       771

Group variable: id                             Number of groups   =       263

                                               Obs per group:
                                                            min =         1
                                                            avg =       2.9
                                                            max =         4

                                               Wald chi2(3)       =    367.14
Log likelihood = -2708.3236                    Prob > chi2        =    0.0000

---------------------------------------------------------------------------
  depression |    Coef.    Std. Err.      z    P>|z|    [95% Conf. Interval]
-------------+-------------------------------------------------------------
        time | -6.350396   .7504495    -8.46   0.000    -7.82125   -4.879542
    time_PST | -4.663613   1.048333    -4.45   0.000    -6.718308  -2.608918
    time_CBT | -5.460471   1.073139    -5.09   0.000    -7.563785  -3.357157
       _cons | 31.69962    .5768601    54.95   0.000    30.56899   32.83024
---------------------------------------------------------------------------


---------------------------------------------------------------------------
  Random-effects Parameters  |   Estimate   Std. Err.    [95% Conf. Interval]
-----------------------------+---------------------------------------------
id: Identity                 |
               var(_cons)    |   46.75738   5.492011     37.14241   58.86136
-----------------------------+---------------------------------------------
               var(Residual) |   40.76049   2.527975     36.09506   46.02896
---------------------------------------------------------------------------
LR test vs. linear model: chibar2(01) = 225.72         Prob >= chibar2 = 0.0000
```

Output 9.6 Results of the alternative repeated measures analysis to estimate the overall intervention effect on average over time in the Internet RCT (PST = problem-solving therapy, CBT = cognitive behavioral therapy)

From the first part of Output 9.5, it can be seen that data from 205 subjects is used in the analysis and that the average number of follow-up measurements is 2.5. In the second part of the output (the fixed part of the model), it can be seen that the regression coefficient for problem-solving therapy (−4.528607) reveals a slightly less strong effect on depression compared to cognitive behavioral therapy (−5.209772). The interpretation of the effect estimates is the difference on average over time in depression between the particular intervention and the waiting list group. These effect estimates are adjusted for the differences at baseline between the groups.

In the alternative repeated measures analysis, the baseline value is not used as covariate, but it is used as outcome. In the model, time and the interaction between the dummy variables for the two interventions and time are added to the model (see Sect. 3.4.2). In this analysis, time is coded 1 for all three follow-up measurements, to obtain an overall treatment effect over time (see Table 3.5). Output 9.6 shows the result of the analysis.

From the first part of Output 9.6, it can be seen that there are 263 subjects included in this analysis instead of the 205 subjects that were included in the longitudinal analysis of covariance reported in Output 9.5. It can further be seen that the maximum number of observations per subject equals 4. This includes the three follow-up measurements and the baseline measurement, because the baseline measurement is part of the output in the alternative repeated measures analysis.

```
Mixed-effects ML regression                    Number of obs      =       682
Group variable: id                             Number of groups   =       263

                                               Obs per group:
                                                          min =          1
                                                          avg =        2.6
                                                          max =          3

                                               Wald chi2(3)       =     110.08
Log likelihood = -2305.4537                    Prob > chi2        =     0.0000

-----------------------------------------------------------------------------
  depression |     Coef.   Std. Err.      z    P>|z|     [95% Conf. Interval]
-------------+---------------------------------------------------------------
intervention |
         PST | -2.465139   1.335626    -1.85   0.065    -5.082918    .152639.
         CBT | -2.098322   1.332211    -1.58   0.115    -4.709408    .512763`
             |
  dep_basel~e |  .7430345    .07274    10.21   0.000     .6004666    .885602:
        _cons |  2.623011   2.514247     1.04   0.297    -2.304824   7.55084!
-----------------------------------------------------------------------------


-----------------------------------------------------------------------------
 Random-effects Parameters  |   Estimate   Std. Err.    [95% Conf. Interval]
----------------------------+------------------------------------------------
id: Identity                |
               var(_cons)   |   68.41501   6.834143      56.25003    83.21086
----------------------------+------------------------------------------------
             var(Residual)  |   21.9512    1.517297      19.16999    25.1359
-----------------------------------------------------------------------------
LR test vs. linear model: chibar2(01) = 390.47       Prob >= chibar2 = 0.0000
```

Output 9.7 Results of the analysis of covariance on the last value carried forward imputed dataset to estimate the overall intervention effect on average over time in the Internet RCT (PST = problem-solving therapy, CBT = cognitive behavioral therapy)

From the second part of Output 9.6, the effect estimates can be obtained. As has been mentioned before, the regression coefficients of the interaction between the two dummy variables for the two interventions and time indicate the effect estimates for the two interventions. So, based on the alternative repeated measures analysis, the effect estimate for problem-solving therapy equals -4.663613 and for cognitive behavioral therapy -5.460471. The interpretation of these effect estimates is the same as for the longitudinal analysis of covariance: the difference in depression on average over time between the particular intervention and the waiting list group.

The alternative repeated measures analysis is a method to include the subjects with only a baseline measurement in the analysis. As has been mentioned before, another option is to impute the missing follow-up measurements. The most simple way to do that is the last value carried forward method. In this case, the available baseline measurement is carried forward to all three follow-up measurements, again assuming no change over time. It should be noted that missing observations in subjects with a baseline measurement but with one or two missing follow-up measurements are not imputed. This is not necessary because (again) mixed model analysis is highly capable of dealing with missing data in the follow-up measurements. Output 9.7 shows the result of the longitudinal analysis of covariance performed on the last value carried forward imputed dataset.

From the first part of Output 9.7, it can be seen that not all missing data is imputed, i.e., not all patients have three follow-up measurements. Only for the

```
Multiple-imputation estimates              Imputations       =        20
Mixed-effects ML regression                Number of obs     =       789

Group variable: id                         Number of groups  =       263
                                           Obs per group:
                                                          min =         3
                                                          avg =       3.0
                                                          max =         3
                                           Average RVI       =    0.4530
                                           Largest FMI       =    0.5149
DF adjustment:    Large sample             DF:           min =     75.34
                                                         avg =    246.73
                                                         max =    445.62
Model F test:      Equal FMI               F(   3,  662.9)   =     21.72
                                           Prob > F          =    0.0000


---------------------------------------------------------------------------
   depression |     Coef.   Std. Err.      t    P>|t|    [95% Conf. Interval]
--------------+------------------------------------------------------------
    condition |
          PST | -4.635601   1.428676   -3.24   0.001    -7.443381  -1.827821
          CBT | -5.045399   1.53039    -3.30   0.001    -8.063378  -2.027419
              |
   dep_basel~e |  .5696981   .0803754    7.09   0.000     .411467    .7279291
        _cons |  7.138994   2.788243    2.56   0.011    1.649431   12.62856
---------------------------------------------------------------------------


---------------------------------------------------------------------------
   Random-effects Parameters  |   Estimate   Std. Err.    [95% Conf. Interval]
-----------------------------+---------------------------------------------
id: Identity                 |
             var(_cons)      |  60.059834   8.220828     47.151844  76.50149
-----------------------------+---------------------------------------------
            var(Residual)    |  31.48487    2.993536     26.454389  37.471942
---------------------------------------------------------------------------
```

Output 9.8 Results of the analysis of covariance on the multiple imputed datasets to estimate the intervention effect on average over time in the Internet RCT (PST = problem-solving therapy, CBT = cognitive behavioral therapy)

58 patients without any follow-up measurement, the missing data are imputed with the last value carried forward imputation method. In the second part of the output, the effect estimates of the two interventions can be obtained. For the problem-solving therapy group, the regression coefficient equals -2.465139, while for the cognitive behavioral therapy group, the regression coefficient equals -2.098322.

As for the situation with one follow-up measurement, also for the situation with more than one follow-up measurement, multiple imputation can be performed to replace the missing data of the follow-up measurements. Also, in this example, predictive mean matching (see Sect. 9.1) was used for the multiple imputation, and also in this example 20 imputed datasets were created, and the imputation model included the baseline value of the outcome and the intervention variable. Output 9.8 shows the result of the pooled longitudinal analysis of covariance performed on the 20 multiple imputed datasets.

From Output 9.8 it can be seen that 20 imputed datasets are used in the analysis. It can also be seen that with the predictive mean matching imputation, all missing values are imputed. So, also the missing observations for the patients with a baseline value but without one or two missing follow-up measurements are imputed. Therefore, all patients have three measurements in the outcome variable. The most

Table 9.4 Overview of the results derived from the different methods

	Effect estimate	95% CI	p-value
Problem-solving therapy			
No imputation	−4.53	−7.33 to −1.73	0.002
Alternative repeated measures	−4.66	−6.72 to −2.61	<0.001
last value carried forward	−2.47	−5.08 to −0.15	0.065
Multiple imputation	−4.64	−7.44 to −1.83	0.001
Cognitive behavioral therapy			
No imputation	−5.21	−8.08 to −2.34	<0.001
Alternative repeated measures	−5.46	−7.56 to −3.36	<0.001
Last value carried forward	−2.10	−4.71 to −0.51	0.115
Multiple imputation	−5.05	−8.06 to −2.03	0.001

interesting part of the output is the second part of the output, which contains the regression coefficients for the two interventions, i.e., the effect estimates. For the problem-solving therapy group, the pooled effect estimate equals −4.635601, while for the cognitive behavioral therapy group, the pooled effect estimate equals −5.045399.

Table 9.4 gives an overview of the results derived from the four analyses performed.

The conclusion of the comparison between the different methods to deal with the problem of missing all follow-up measurements when the baseline value is available is more or less the same in RCTs with one follow-up measurement as in RCTs with more than one follow-up measurement. Although the results obtained from the longitudinal analysis of covariance in this situation are comparable to the ones obtained from the alternative repeated measures analysis and the multiple imputation, the effect estimates obtained from the analysis of covariance performed on the last value carried forward imputation method were again remarkably lower than the effect estimates obtained from the other three methods. From the baseline value carried forward method, it is often suggested that it leads to a conservative estimation of the intervention effect (which is the case in the examples used in this chapter) and is therefore an acceptable method to analyze RCT data. That the last value carried forward imputation method leads to an underestimation of the intervention effect is, however, not always true but depends highly on the setting of the study. Suppose, an intervention is performed to reduce the decline in physical functioning in elderly people; the baseline value carried forward assumes no decline, which is actually a positive result. When, on the other hand, an intervention is performed to reduce blood pressure, as in the first example, the baseline value carried forward assuming no reduction can be classified as a negative result.

From Table 9.4 it can also be seen that the 95% confidence interval around the effect estimates for the alternative repeated measures analysis is a bit smaller than the ones obtained from the longitudinal analysis of covariance on the non-imputed data and on the multiple imputed data. This smaller 95% confidence interval is caused by the fact that the alternative repeated measures analysis uses more observations in the outcome variable, which leads to slightly smaller standard errors (see Sect. 3.5). The multiple imputed datasets are also full datasets, but because the standard error of the pooled effect estimates also contain the uncertainty of the imputations, the standard error is increased. This leads to broader (more valid) 95% confidence intervals.

9.3 Comments

9.3.1 Sensitivity Analysis

In this chapter, different methods to deal with the problem of missing all follow-up measurements in an RCT while the baseline value of the outcome is available were compared with each other. In the examples the missing follow-up data was (highly) related to the baseline value. Nevertheless, the effect estimates of the (longitudinal) analysis of covariance on the non-imputed data, the alternative mixed model analyses, and the (longitudinal) analysis of covariance on the multiple imputed data were only slightly different. Because it is not clear which of the effect estimates indicates the real intervention effect, it is suggested that sensitivity analyses should be included in the analysis of RCT data in order to obtain a more robust effect estimate (European Medicines Agency, 2010). Surprisingly, the results of sensitivity analyses on RCT data are almost never reported in the scientific literature, and when they are reported, they are mostly performed to show the robustness of the analysis against different assumptions underlying the statistical analysis. However, sensitivity analyses can also be performed with different statistical methods. Based on the examples in this chapter, it seems to be appropriate to report the results of different statistical methods as sensitivity analyses, especially in situations where the number of subjects with a baseline value but without follow-up measurements is relatively high.

9.3.2 Selective Imputation

It is sometimes argued that a selective imputation method should be applied in the situation when a baseline value is available but all follow-up measurements are missing (European Medicines Agency, 2010). To use a selective imputation method, however, some additional information must be available. This additional information includes whether a subject who is randomized into the intervention group, with a baseline value but without follow-up measurements, actually received the intervention. The general idea is that when these subjects did not receive the intervention, selective imputation can be used in which data of these subjects were imputed as if they belong to the control condition. It should be realized that selective imputation can only be applied in situations where it is known whether the subjects actually received the intervention or not. When this information is available, this selective imputation seems to be an acceptable approach (European Medicines Agency, 2010). However, it is questionable whether or not the analysis with selective imputation can be classified as intention-to-treat. In the selective imputation method, the subjects in the intervention group with missing data were imputed as if they were allocated to the control condition. And although the analysis is on an intention-to-treat basis, the imputation is not. On the other hand, when it is ignored that the subjects with missing data at the follow-up measurements did not receive the intervention, the effect estimates were highly overestimated (Twisk et al., 2020). An overestimation of the effect estimate is not what you may expect from an intention-to-treat analysis. It should also be realized that a potential limitation of selective imputation is the fact that the subjects who did not receive the intervention were imputed as they belong to the control condition. It is however questionable whether that is correct, because in the literature there are some examples showing that not adhering the intervention is different from belonging to the control condition (Murray et al., 2020; Wilson, 2010). So therefore, the results of the analyses with a selective imputation method can be slightly invalid and should be interpreted with caution.

9.3.3 Other Comments

In this chapter, different methods were used to analyze RCT data in which subjects had a baseline value but missed all follow-up measurements. Although less common, it is also possible that subjects were not measured at baseline but do have follow-up measurements. In an analysis adjusted for the baseline value, these subjects are (of course) also excluded from the analysis. It is expected that the probability of having a missing baseline value is not related to the follow-up measurements, so this situation can be considered as missing completely at random (MCAR). When this is the case, regular mixed model analysis, alternative mixed model analysis, and multiple imputation will not lead to very different effect estimates. Also because the percentage of subjects without a baseline value but with follow-up measurements, in general, will be relatively low.

It should be noted that the assumption of using either mixed model analysis or multiple imputation is that the missing data is at random (MAR). In real-life data, MCAR and MAR are probably the most common; however, missing data can also be not at random (MNAR). Although it is not possible to evaluate whether missing data is MNAR or MAR, there are methods available that claim to appropriately take into account missing data which is MNAR. These methods, such as pattern mixture models, selection models, and shared parameter models (Fiero et al., 2017; Little, 1993, 1994; Molenberghs & Kenward, 2007; Tsonaka et al., 2009), are complicated and difficult to interpret and, therefore, not often used in practice. It should also be noted that in the examples used in this chapter, only the baseline value and the intervention variable were used for the imputation models. Although it is possible that missingness is related to other variables, the baseline value of the outcome is (mostly) by far the best predictor of the missing outcomes at the follow-up measurements. So, adding other variables to the imputation models would not add much information to the imputation models and would therefore probably not change the results of the examples discussed in this chapter.

9.4   Recommendation

When, in an RCT, the baseline value is available and all follow-up measurements are missing, it is not necessary to use (multiple) imputation. Using an analysis of covariance on the available data or the alternative repeated measures analysis will provide more than acceptable effect estimates.

Chapter 10
Sample Size Calculations

10.1 Introduction

Before performing an RCT, most researchers believe that it is necessary to calculate the number of subjects that are needed in the RCT to make sure that a predefined effect will be statistically significant. It is necessary because sample size calculations are a prerequisite for research grants and must be submitted to (medical) ethics committees. Furthermore, for medical studies, sample size calculations are part of the so-called CONSORT statement. This means that, without a sample size calculation, a paper reporting the results of a medical RCT will not be published in any of the major (medical) journals. It should be realized that the importance of sample size calculations is highly questionable. First, sample size calculations are based on many assumptions, which can easily be changed, and in which case the number of subjects needed will be totally different. Second, sample size calculations are based on testing theory (i.e., statistical testing and statistical significance). This is rather strange, because recently the importance of testing theory is becoming more and more questionable. Nevertheless, many people believe in the importance of sample size calculations.

Basically sample size calculation formulas are developed to calculate the number of subjects needed in an RCT to get a certain difference between the intervention and control groups statistically significant. In the standard sample size calculation formula, this difference is the difference at one follow-up measurement. For continuous outcome variables, the standard sample size calculation formula (Eq. 10.1) can be used:

$$N_1 = \frac{\left(Z_{(1-\alpha/2)} + Z_{(1-\beta)}\right)^2 \times \sigma^2 \times (r+1)}{v^2 \times r} \tag{10.1}$$

where N_1 = sample size for the intervention group, α = significance level, $Z_{(1-\alpha/2)} = (1 - \alpha/2)$ percentile point of the standard normal distribution, $(1 - \beta)$ = power,

© The Author(s), under exclusive license to Springer Nature Switzerland AG 2021
J. W. R. Twisk, *Analysis of Data from Randomized Controlled Trials*,
https://doi.org/10.1007/978-3-030-81865-4_10

$Z_{(1-\beta)} = (1 - \beta)$ percentile point of the standard normal distribution, $\sigma =$ standard deviation of the outcome variable, and $r =$ ratio of the number of subjects in the groups to be compared, i.e., N_0/N_1, where $N_0 =$ sample size for the control group and $v =$ difference in mean value of the outcome variable between the groups.

For dichotomous outcome variables, a comparable sample size calculation formula can be used (Eqs. 10.2a, 10.2b):

$$N_1 = \frac{\left(Z_{(1-\alpha_2)} + Z_{(1-\beta)}\right)^2 \times \bar{p}(1-\bar{p}) \times (r+1)}{(p_1 - p_0)^2 \times r} \qquad (10.2a)$$

$$\bar{p} = \frac{p_1 + (r \times p_0)}{1 + r} \qquad (10.2b)$$

where $N_1 =$ sample size for the intervention group, $\alpha =$ significance level, $Z_{(1-\alpha/2)} = (1-\alpha/2)$ percentile point of the standard normal distribution, $(1 - \beta) =$ power, $Z_{(1 - \beta)} = (1 - \beta)$ percentile point of the standard normal distribution, $\bar{p} =$ average of p_0, and p_1, $r =$ ratio of the number of subjects in the groups to be compared, i.e., N_0/N_1 where $N_0 =$ sample size for the control group, $p_1 =$ proportion of cases in the intervention group, and $p_0 =$ proportion of cases in the control group.

When a cluster RCT is performed (see Chap. 4), the sample size needs to be adjusted to take into account the dependency of the observations within the cluster. Because of that dependency, more subjects are needed than calculated with a standard sample size calculation formula (Twisk, 2018). There are different ways to calculate the adjusted sample size. Equation (10.3) shows the first correction factor, which is known as the conservative correction factor:

$$m \times n = N \times [1 + (n - 1)\rho] \qquad (10.3)$$

where $N =$ number of subjects calculated with the standard sample size calculation formula, $m =$ number of clusters (e.g., number of hospitals, nursery homes, medical doctors, schools, families, etc.), $n =$ number of observations within each cluster, and $\rho =$ intraclass correlation coefficient (ICC).

It is also possible to calculate the relative effectiveness of a certain sample size, when that sample size is applied in a cluster RCT (Eq. 10.4):

$$N_{effective} = \frac{N}{[1 + (n - 1)\rho]} \qquad (10.4)$$

where $N_{effective} =$ effective sample size by a given standard sample size (based on m times n observations).

Equation (10.5) shows the second correction factor that can be used to calculate the required sample size for a cluster RCT. This correction factor is known as the liberal correction factor. Equation (10.6) shows the corresponding equation to calculate the effective sample size:

$$m = \frac{N}{1 + (n - 1)(1 - \rho)} \tag{10.5}$$

where N = number of subjects calculated with the standard sample size calculation formula, m = number of clusters (e.g., number of hospitals, nursery homes, medical doctors, schools, families, etc.), n = number of observations for each cluster, and ρ = intraclass correlation coefficient (ICC):

$$N_{\text{effective}} = m \times [1 + (n - 1)\rho] \tag{10.6}$$

where $N_{\text{effective}}$ = effective sample size by a given standard sample size (based on m times n observations).

In many situations, however, a more simple adjustment formula is used. In this simple adjustment, the sample size calculated with the standard sample size calculation formula is multiplied by the 100 + intraclass correlation coefficient (ICC) percentage. So, when the ICC is assumed to be 0.10, the standard sample size (i.e., the one calculated with the standard sample size calculation formula) is multiplied by 110%, etc.

When more than one follow-up measurement is performed, the sample size needs to be further adjusted to take into account the dependency of the repeated observations within the subject. Because of that dependency, less subjects are needed than calculated with a standard sample size calculation formula (Twisk, 2013). Equation (10.7) shows the multiplication factor for an RCT with more than one follow-up measurement:

$$\frac{\{1 + (T - 1) \times \rho\}}{T} \tag{10.7}$$

where T = number of follow-up measurements and ρ = correlation coefficient between the repeated measurements.

When a cluster RCT with more than one follow-up measurement is performed, the situation is slightly more complex. In that situation, there are two dependencies to take into account: (1) the dependency of the observations within in a cluster, which requires a bigger sample size, and (2) the dependency of the repeated observations within the subject, which requires a smaller sample size. Both should be taken into account to calculate the required sample size. The same situation more or less occurs in a stepped wedge trial (see Chap. 6). When a sample size must be calculated for a stepped wedge trial, also both dependencies must be taken into account (Baio et al., 2015; Hemming & Taljaard, 2016; Woertman et al., 2013).

10.2 Example

As has been mentioned before, the calculation of the required sample size is based on many assumptions. Table 10.1 shows the assumptions of a cluster RCT with more than one follow-up measurement performed within general practitioner (GPs) with the aim to reduce systolic blood pressure.

The first step in the sample size calculation is to apply the standard sample size calculation formula (see Eq. 10.1):

$$N_1 = \frac{7.85 \times 10^2 \times 2}{5^2} = 62.8$$

So, with 62.8 subjects, a difference of 5 mmHg will be statistically significant with a significance level of 0.05 and a power of 80%, assuming a standard deviation of 15 mmHg. When this number is calculated, it is a sort of common practice to take into account the fact that some of the subjects will drop out during the study, and because of that, the required sample size is slightly increased. In this case the sample size per group can be increased to 70 subjects, assuming a drop out percentage of around 10%.

In the next step, the clustering of the observations within the GP must be taken into account, and it is assumed that this correlation equals 0.1 (see Table 10.1). To do this, for instance, Eq. (10.3) can be applied. Because there is a fixed number of 20 GPs available, the number of subjects within a GP will be 7:

$$m \times n = 70 \times [1 + (7 - 1) \times 0.1] = 112$$

So, instead of 70 subjects per group, when taking into account the clustering of the subject observations within the GP, 112 subjects per group are needed.

In the next step, it must be taken into account that there are two follow-up measurements and that there is an assumed correlation of 0.6 between the two follow-up measurements within the subject (see Table 10.1). To do that, Eq. (10.7) can be applied to obtain the multiplication factor:

Table 10.1 Assumptions for the sample size calculation of a cluster RCT

Number of follow-up measurements	2
Average difference to be detected	5 mmHg
Assumed standard deviation	10 mmHg
Assumed correlation between repeated measures	0.6
Assumed correlation between gps	0.1
Number of GPs	20
Power	80%
Significance	0.05
Ratio of the number of observations in the groups to be compared	1

$$\frac{\{1 + (2 - 1) \times 0.6\}}{2} = 0.8$$

$$0.8 \times 112 = 89.6$$

So, taken into account the fact that there are two follow-up measurements with a correlation within the subject of 0.6, the number of subjects needed in this cluster RCT reduces to around 90 subjects per group. So for each GP around nine subjects should be included in this cluster RCT with two follow-up measurements.

10.3 Comments

It is obvious that the number of subjects needed in a trial like this highly depends on the assumptions made. A slightly higher correlation between the subjects within the GP will increase the required sample size considerably. The same holds for a higher correlation between the two follow-up measurements within the subject, a higher standard deviation, and a lower expected difference between the intervention group and the control group. Also when a power of 90% is used, the required sample size will increase. In fact, changing the assumptions only a bit can have a huge influence on the results of the sample size calculation.

The problem with sample size calculations is that nobody knows what the numbers will be in the study to be performed. So, basically, each sample size calculation will be a (wild) guess and should, therefore, be interpreted with great caution. Or even better, sample size calculations should not be done at all. Other arguments, such as logistic, financial, and ethical considerations can better be used to define the required sample size for an RCT.

Chapter 11
Miscellaneous

11.1 Different Designs

In the foregoing chapters, several RCT designs were discussed: a regular RCT with one follow-up measurement (Chap. 2), a regular RCT with more than one follow-up measurement (Chap. 3), a cluster RCT (Chap. 4), a cross-over trial (Chap. 5), a stepped wedge trial (Chap. 6), and (a series of) n-of-1 trials (Chap. 7). In most of these designs, a baseline measurement is performed to obtain an estimation of the outcome variable before the start of the intervention. This baseline measurement provides the possibility to adjust for the differences in the outcome variable at baseline between the groups. It is, however, also possible that the baseline measurement itself has an influence on the outcome variable. This is known as a test or learning effect. In a Solomon four-group design, two groups are allocated to the intervention in which for one group a baseline measurement is performed, and for the other group not. The same procedure is applied to the control group. By comparing the effect estimates of the four groups, test or learning effects can be detected.

In some RCTs, multiple baseline measurements are performed. The general idea behind these multiple baseline measurements is to obtain a more robust estimation of the baseline value. In that situation, mostly the average value of the multiple baseline measurements is calculated, and this average is used as baseline measurement in the analysis. However, looking at the stepped wedge trial (see Chap. 6) and the example in the series of n-of-trials (see Chap. 7), there are also multiple baseline measurements for some or all of the randomized subjects. In the analyses, however, not the average value of the baseline measurements was used for the analysis, but all measurements were used in the mixed model analysis taken into account the correlation between the repeated observations within the subject. Although this is of course also possible in regular RCTs with more than one baseline measurement, it is not much used in practice.

© The Author(s), under exclusive license to Springer Nature Switzerland AG 2021   157
J. W. R. Twisk, *Analysis of Data from Randomized Controlled Trials*,
https://doi.org/10.1007/978-3-030-81865-4_11

11.2   Statistical Testing of Baseline Differences in an RCT

It is often argued that an adjustment for the baseline difference in the outcome variable in an RCT is only necessary when the difference between the groups is statistically significant. This is, however, a huge misunderstanding. Basically, the baseline value of the outcome variable can be seen as a confounder in the estimation of the intervention effect. A variable is considered to be a confounder when it is related to both the independent and the dependent variable in the statistical model. Because in an RCT, the baseline value of the outcome is highly related to the outcome at the follow-up measurement(s), even a small difference in the baseline value of the outcome between the two groups can have a (strong) confounding effect. It is, therefore, advised always to adjust for the baseline value of the outcome variable irrespective whether the difference is significant or not. Furthermore, it should be realized that statistical significance does not say anything about the magnitude of a particular difference and also not about the influence of the differences between the baseline values on the estimated intervention effect.

The issue of testing for statistical significance also holds for the adjustment for other covariates. Although the adjustment for other covariates is less important than the adjustment for the baseline value of the outcome, it can still be important to consider adjustment for other covariates (Kahan, 2014). When a covariate is related to the outcome and when that covariate differs between the two groups, the particular covariate is considered to be a confounder in the estimation of the intervention effect. Again, note that it is not necessary that the covariate is significantly related to the outcome or that the covariate is significantly different between the two groups. Significance does not play an important role in the amount of confounding the particular covariate has. Although many researchers believe that it has to be done, it is, therefore, of no use to statistically test for baseline differences between the intervention and the control group. Luckily, this testing nonsense has been noticed by other authors as well (de Boer et al., 2015; Petterson et al., 2017).

11.3   Analyzing Within-Group Changes in an RCT

When data from an RCT is analyzed, the effect of the intervention can be estimated by comparing the outcome variable between the intervention group and the control group. In many publications, however, there is also an estimation of the within-group changes over time. This is especially the case when there is no significant intervention effect. Although it is not wrong to estimate the within-group changes over time, the interpretation of the within-group changes can lead to wrong conclusions about the effectiveness of an intervention.

11.3.1   Example

The example dataset is an RCT with one follow-up measurement aiming to reduce systolic blood pressure. Table 11.1 shows the descriptive information of this study.

In Table 11.1 it can be seen that in the intervention group there is a decrease in systolic blood pressure over time and that there is also a decrease in systolic blood pressure in the control group. However, the decrease in systolic blood pressure in the intervention group is more pronounced than the decrease in systolic blood pressure in the control group. So, the intervention group is performing slightly better than the control group. Furthermore, it can be seen that there is only a small difference in the baseline systolic blood pressure values between the two groups.

Output 11.1 shows the results of the analysis of covariance performed to estimate the effect of the intervention. As has been mentioned before (see Chap. 2), in the analysis of covariance, blood pressure measured at the follow-up measurement is used as the outcome variable. The intervention variable is used as independent variable, while the baseline measure of systolic blood pressure is added to the model as covariate.

From Output 11.1 it can be seen that the regression coefficient for the intervention variable equals -1.2744, which indicates that in the intervention group, the systolic blood pressure at the follow-up measurement is 1.2744 mmHg lower than in the control group. This difference between the groups is adjusted for the (small) baseline differences between the groups. Besides the intervention effect, the output also shows the 95% confidence interval around the intervention effect (ranging from -4.746889 to 1.198089) and the corresponding p-value, which is 0.469. This p-value indicates that the effect of the intervention is not statistically significant.

Table 11.1 Mean and standard deviation (between brackets) of systolic blood pressure regarding the example RCT

	Baseline	Follow-up measurement
Intervention ($N = 59$)	130.8 (11.8)	127.2 (12.0)
Control ($N = 60$)	130.4 (17.1)	128.2 (13.6)

```
      Source |       SS           df       MS            Number of obs   =         119
-------------+----------------------------------         F(2, 116)       =       47.68
       Model |  8716.41006         2   4358.20503        Prob > F        =      0.0000
    Residual |  10603.4387       116   91.4089541        R-squared       =      0.4512
-------------+----------------------------------         Adj R-squared   =      0.4417
       Total |  19319.8487       118   163.727532        Root MSE        =      9.5608

------------------------------------------------------------------------------
       syst1 |      Coef.   Std. Err.      t    P>|t|     [95% Conf. Interval]
-------------+----------------------------------------------------------------
intervention |    -1.2744   1.753228    -0.73   0.469    -4.746889    2.198089
    baseline |   .5865899   .0601656     9.75   0.000     .4674244    .7057553
       _cons |   51.73801   7.939117     6.52   0.000     36.01359    67.46243
------------------------------------------------------------------------------
```

Output 11.1 Results of the analysis of covariance to estimate the effect of the intervention

```
    Source |       SS           df       MS            Number of obs   =        59
-----------+------------------------------------       F(0, 58)        =      0.00
     Model |        0            0        .            Prob > F        =        .
  Residual |   7773.52542       58    134.0263         R-squared       =    0.0000
-----------+------------------------------------       Adj R-squared   =    0.0000
     Total |   7773.52542       58    134.0263         Root MSE        =    11.577

--------------------------------------------------------------------------------
    change |     Coef.    Std. Err.       t     P>|t|     [95% Conf. Interval]
-----------+--------------------------------------------------------------------
     _cons |  -3.644068   1.507193     -2.42   0.019    -6.661043   -.6270922
--------------------------------------------------------------------------------
```

Output 11.2 Result of the intercept-only linear regression analysis to obtain the within-group change for the intervention group

```
    Source |       SS           df       MS            Number of obs   =        60
-----------+------------------------------------       F(0, 59)        =      0.00
     Model |        0            0        .            Prob > F        =        .
  Residual |    7145.65        59    121.112712        R-squared       =    0.0000
-----------+------------------------------------       Adj R-squared   =    0.0000
     Total |    7145.65        59    121.112712        Root MSE        =    11.005

--------------------------------------------------------------------------------
    change |     Coef.    Std. Err.       t     P>|t|     [95% Conf. Interval]
-----------+--------------------------------------------------------------------
     _cons |     -2.15    1.420755     -1.51   0.136    -4.992924    .6929245
--------------------------------------------------------------------------------
```

Output 11.3 Result of the intercept-only linear regression analysis to obtain the within-group change for the control group

To analyze the within-group change, first, the change scores have to be calculated, and, second, the change scores have to be analyzed for each group separately. To get an estimate of the within-group change for both the intervention and the control group, two intercept-only linear regression analyses must be performed. The estimate of the intercept in an intercept-only model is the estimate of the within-group change.

Outputs 11.2 and 11.3 show the results of the two intercept-only linear regression analyses for the intervention group and the control group, respectively.

In Output 11.2 it can be seen that the intercept value for the intervention group equals -3.644068, which indicates that the systolic blood pressure at the follow-up measurement is 3.644 mmHg lower compared to the baseline measurement. It can further be seen that the corresponding p-value equals 0.019, which indicates that there is a significant change over time in the intervention group. In Output 11.3 it can be seen that the intercept value for the control group equals -2.15, which indicates that for the control group the systolic blood pressure at the follow-up measurement is 2.15 mmHg lower at the follow-up measurement compared to the baseline measurement. The key issue here is that the change over time in the control group is not statistically significant (the p-value $= 0.136$).

Although the analyses are not wrong, many researchers combine the two results of the analyses regarding the within-group changes into a wrong conclusion. They argue that there is a significant intervention effect because there is a significant change in the intervention group, while there is nonsignificant change in the control group. From the results of the analysis of covariance reported in Output 11.1, however, it was already concluded that there was no significant difference between the groups. So, although the analysis of the within-group changes is not wrong per se, it is important to realize that it is not correct to draw conclusions regarding intervention effects based on the significance or non-significance of the within-group changes.

References

Albert, P. S. (1999). Longitudinal data analysis (repeated measures) in clinical trials. *Statistics in Medicine, 18*, 1707–1732.

Apeldoorn, A. T., Ostelo, R. W., van Helvoirt, H., Fritz, J. M., Knol, D. L., van Tulder, M., & de Vet, H. (2012). A randomized controlled trial on the effectiveness of a classification-based system for subacute and chronic low back pain. *Spine, 37*, 1347–1356.

Baio, G., Copas, A., Ambler, G., Hargreaveas, J., Beard, E., & Omar, R. Z. (2015). Sample size calculation for a stepped wedge trial. *Trials, 16*, 354.

Bellamy, S. L., Gibberd, R., Hancock, L., Howley, P., Kennedy, B., Klar, N., Lipsitz, S., & Ryan, L. (2009). Analysis of dichotomous outcome data for community intervention studies. *Statistical Methods in Medical Research, 9*, 135.

Blomquist, N. (1977). On the relation between change and initial value. *Journal of the American Statistical Association, 72*, 746–749.

Box, G. E. P., & Jenkins, G. M. (1994). *Time series analysis, forecasting and control* (3rd ed.). Prentice Hall.

Brown, C. A., & Lilford, R. J. (2006). The stepped wedge trial design: A systematic review. *BMC Medical Research Methodology, 6*, 54.

Chen, X., & Chen, P. (2014). A comparison of four methods for the analysis of N-of-1 trials. *PLoS ONE, 9*(2), e87752. https://doi.org/10.1371/journal.pone.0087752

de Boer, M. R., Waterlander, W. E., Kuijper, L. D., Steenhuis, I. H., & Twisk, J. W. (2015). Testing for baseline differences in randomized controlled trials: An unhealthy research behavior that is hard to eradicate. *International Journal of Behavioral Nutrition and Physical Activity, 24*, 4.

European Medicines Agency. (2010). Guideline on missing data in confirmatory clinical trials. https://www.ema.europa.eu/documents/scientific-guideline/guideline-missing-data-confirmatory-clinical-trials_en.pdf)

Fiero, M. H., Hsu, C.-H., & Bell, M. L. (2017). A pattern-mixture model approach for handling missing continuous outcome data in longitudinal cluster randomized trials. *Statistics in Medicine, 36*, 4094–4105.

Fitzmaurice, G.M., Laird, N.M. and Ware, J.H. (2004) Applied longitudinal data analysis. ,

Forbes, A. B., & Carlin, J. B. (2005). "Residual change" analysis is not equivalent to analysis of covariance. *Journal of Clinical Epidemiology, 58*, 540–541.

Goldstein, H. (2003). *Multilevel statistical models* (3nd ed.). Edward Arnold.

Gravel, J., Opatrny, L., & Shapiro, S. (2007). The intention-to-treat approach in randomized controlled trials: Are authors saying what they do and doing what they say? *Clinical Trials, 4*, 350–356.

Greenland, S., & Robins, J. M. (2009). Identifiability, exchangeability and confounding revisited. *Epidemiologic Perspectives & Innovations, 6*, 4.

Hemming, K., & Taljaard, M. (2016). Sample size calculations for stepped wedge and cluster randomised trials: A unified approach. *Journal of Clinical Epidemiology, 69*, 137–146.

Heo, M., & Leon, A. C. (2005). Comparison of statistical methods for analysis of clustered binary outcomes. *Statistics in Medicine, 24*, 911–923.

Hernan, M. A., Clayton, D., & Keiding, N. (2011). The Simpson's paradox unravelled. *International Journal of Epidemiology, 40*, 780–785.

Hollis, S., & Campbell, F. (1999). What is meant by intention-to-treat analysis? Survey of published randomized controlled trials. *BMJ, 319*, 670–674.

Hu, F. B., Goldberg, J., Hedeker, D., Flay, B. R., & Pentz, M. (1998). Comparison of population-averaged and subject-specific approaches for analyzing repeated binary outcomes. *American Journal of Epidemiology, 147*, 694–703.

Hubbard, A. E., Ahern, J., Fleischer, N. L., van der Laan, M., Lippman, S. A., Jewell, N., Bruckner, T., & Satariano, W. A. (2010). To GEE or not to GEE. Comparing population average and mixed models for estimating the associations between neighborhood risk factors and health. *Epidemiology, 21*, 467–474.

Hussey, M. A., & Hughes, J. P. (2007). Design and analysis if stepped wedge cluster randomised trials. *Contemporary Clinical Trials, 28*, 182–191.

Kahan, B. C. (2014). The risk and rewards of covariate adjustment in randomized trials: An assessment of 12 outcomes from 8 studies. *Trials, 15*, 139.

Kennedy-Schaffer, L., de Gruttola, V., & Lipsitch, M. (2019). Novel methods for the analysis of stepped wedge cluster randomized trials. *Statistics in Medicine*, 1–30.

Kenward, M. G., & Jones, B. (2008). *Design and analysis of cross-over-trials: Handbook of statistics* (Vol. 27). Elsevier.

Kim, H.-Y., Preisser, J. S., Rozier, R. G., & Valiyaparambi, J. V. (2006). Multilevel analysis of group randomized trials with binary data. *Community Dentistry and Oral Epidemiology, 34*, 241–251.

Kotz, D., Spigt, M., Arts, I. C. W., Crutzen, R., & Viechtbauer, W. (2012). Use of the stepped wedge design cannot be recommended: A critical appraisal and comparison with the classic cluster randomised controlled trial design. *Journal of Clinical Epidemiology, 65*, 1249–1252.

Laird, N. M., & Ware, J. H. (1982). Random effects models for longitudinal data. *Biometrics, 38*, 963–974.

Lesaffre, E., & Spiessens, B. (2001). On the effect of the number of quadrature points in a logistic random-effects model: An example. *Applied Statistics, 50*, 325–335.

Liang, K., & Zeger, S. L. (1986). Longitudinal data analysis using generalized linear models. *Biometrika, 73*, 45–51.

Liang, K-Y., Zeger, S.L. (1993). Regression analysis for correlated data. *Annual Review of Public Health*, 14, 43-68.

Lillie, E. O., Patay, B., Diamant, J., Issell, B., Topol, E. J., & Schork, N. J. (2011). The n-of-1 clinical trial: The ultimate strategy for individualizing medicine? *Personalized Medicine, 8*, 161–173.

Little, R. J. A. (1993). Pattern-mixture models for multivariate incomplete data. *Journal of the American Statistical Association, 88*, 125–134.

Little, R. J. A. (1994). A class of pattern-mixture models for normal incomplete data. *Biometrika, 81*, 471–483.

Little, R. J. A. (1995). Modelling the drop-out mechanism repeated measures studies. *Journal of the American Statistical Association, 90*, 1112–1121.

Liu, Q., & Pierce, D. A. (1994). A note on Gauss–Hermite quadrature. *Biometrika, 81*, 624–629.

McCleary, R., & Hay, R. A. (1980). *Applied time series analysis for the social sciences*. Sage.

Mdege, N. D., Man, M.-S., Taylor, C. A., & Torgerson, D. J. (2011). Systematic review of stepped wedge cluster randomized trials shows that design is particularly used to evaluate interventions during routine implementation. *Journal of Clinical Epidemiology, 64*, 936–948.

Molenberghs, G., & Kenward, M. G. (2007). *Missing data in clinical studies*. Wiley.

Morris, T. P., White, I. R., & Royston, P. (2014). Tuning multiple imputation by predictive mean matching and local residual draws. *BMC Medical Research Methodology, 14*, 75–87.

Mukaka, M., White, S. A., Terlouw, D. J., Mwapasa, V., & Kalilani-Phiri, L. (2016). Is using multiple imputation better than a complete case analysis for estimating a prevalence (risk) difference in randomized controlled trials when binary outcome observations are missing. *Trials, 17*, 341.

Muntinga, M. E., Hoogendijk, E. O., van Leeuwen, K. M., van Hout, H. P. J., Twisk, J. W. R., van der Horst, H. E., Nijpels, G., & Jansen, A. P. D. (2012). Implementing the chronic care model for frail older adults in the Netherlands: Study protocol of ACT (frail older adults: Care in transition). *BMC Geriatrics, 12*, 19.

Murray, E. J., Claggett, B. L., Granger, B., & Solomon, S. D. (2020). Adherence-adjustment in placebo-controlled randomized trials: An application to the candesartan in heart faillure randomized trial. *Contemporary Clinical Trials, 90*, 105937.

Newman, S. C. (2004). Commonalities in the classical, collapsibility and counterfactual concepts in confounding. *Journal of Clinical Epidemiology, 57*, 325–329.

Omar, R. Z., Wright, E. M., Turner, R. M., & Thompson, S. G. (1999). Analysing repeated measurements data: A practical comparison of methods. *Statistics in Medicine, 18*, 1587–1603.

Peixeiro, M., (2019). *The complete guide to time series analysis and forecasting understand moving average, exponential smoothing, stationarity, autocorrelation, SARIMA, and apply these techniques in two projects*. https://towardsdatascience.com/

Petterson, R. L., Tran, M., Koffel, J., & Stovitz, S. D. (2017). Statistical testing of baseline differences in sports medicine RCT's: A systematic evaluation. *BMJ Open Sport & Exercise Medicine, 3*.

Proper, K. I., Koning, M., Beek, A., van der Hildebrandt, V. H., Bosscher, R. J., & van Mechelen, W. (2003). The effectiveness of worksite physical activity programms on physical activity, physiscal fitness, and healt. *Clinical Journal of Sports Medicine, 13*, 106–117.

Rabe-Hesketh, S., & Skrondal, A. (2001). Parameterisation of multivariate random effects models for categorical data. *Biometrics, 57*, 1256–1264.

Rothman, K. J., & Greenland, S. (1998). *Modern Epidemiology*. Lippincott-Raven Publishers.

StataCorp. (2017). *Stata Statistical Software: Release 15*. StataCorp LLC.

Subramanian, S. V. (2004). The relevance of multilevel statistical methods for identifying causal neighbourhood effects. *Social Science & Medicine, 58*, 1961–1967.

ten Have, T. R., Ratcliffe, S. J., Reboussin, B. A., & Miller, M. E. (2004). Deviations from the population-average cluster-specific relationship for clustered binary data. *Statistical Methods in Medical Research, 13*, 3–16.

Thompson, J. A., Davey, C., Fielding, K., Hargreaves, J. R., & Hayes, R. J. (2018). Robust analysis of stepped wedge trials using cluster level summaries within periods. *Statistics in Medicine, 37*, 2487–2500.

Tsonaka, R., Verbeke, G., & Lesaffre, E. (2009). A semi-parametric shared parameter model to handle nonmonotone nonignorable missingness. *Biometrics, 65*, 81–87.

Twisk, J. (2004). Longitudinal data analysis. A comparison between generalized estimating equations and random coefficient analysis. *European Journal of Epidemiology, 19*, 769–776.

Twisk, J. (2018). *Applied mixed model analysis*. Cambridge University Press.

Twisk, J., Bosman, L., Hoekstra, T., Rijnhart, J., Welten, M., & Heymans, M. (2018). Different ways to estimate treatment effects in randomised controlled trials. *Contemporary Clinical Trials Communications, 10*, 80–85.

Twisk, J., de Boer, M., de Vente, W., & Heymans, M. (2013). Multiple imputation of missing values was not necessary before performing a longitudinal mixed-model analysis. *Journal of Clinical Epidemiology, 66*, 1022–1028.

Twisk, J., & Proper, K. (2004). Evaluation of the results of a randomized controlled trial: How to define changes between baseline and follow-up. *Journal of Clinical Epidemiology, 57*, 223–228.

Twisk, J. W., & de Vente, W. (2008). The analysis of randomised controlled data with more than one follow-up measurement. A comparison between different approaches. *European Journal of Epidemiology, 23*, 655–660.

Twisk, J. W., Hoogendijk, E. O., Zwijsen, S. A., & de Boer, M. R. (2016). Different methods to analyze stepped wedge trial designs revealed different aspects of intervention effects. *Journal of Clinical Epidemiology, 72*, 75–83.

Twisk, J. W. R. (2006). *Applied multilevel analysis. A practical guide.* Cambridge University Press.

Twisk, J. W. R. (2013). *Applied longitudinal data analysis for epidemiology* (2nd ed.). Cambridge University Press.

Twisk, J. W. R., & de Vente, W. (2019). Hybrid models were found to be very elegant to disentangle longitudinal within- and between-subject relationships. *Journal of Clinical Epidemiology, 107*, 66–70.

Twisk, J. W. R., de Vente, W., Apeldoorn, A. T., & de Boer, M. (2017). Should we use logistic mixed model analysis for the effect estimation in a longitudinal RCT with a dichotomous outcome variable? *Epidemiology, Biostatistics and Public Health, 14*(3), 1–8.

Twisk, J. W. R., Rijnhart, J. M., Hoekstra, T., Schuster, N. A., ter Wee, M. M., & Heymans, M. W. (2020). Intention-to-treat analysis when only a baseline value is available. *Contemporary Clinical Trials Communications, 20*, 100684.

Twisk, J. W. R., Smidt, N., & de Vente, W. (2005). Applied analysis of recurrent events: A practical overview. *Journal of Epidemiology and Community Health, 59*, 706–710.

van Buuren, S. (2007). Multiple imputation of discrete and continuous data by fully conditional specification. *Statistical Methods in Medical Research, 16*, 219–242.

van Dijk, R. A., Rauwerda, J. A., Steyn, M., Twisk, J. W., & Stehouwer, C. D. (2001). Long-term homocysteine-lowering treatment with folic acid plus pyridoxine is associated with decreased blood pressure but not with improved brachial artery endothelium-dependent vasodilation or carotid artery stiffness: A 2-year, randomized, placebo-controlled trial. *Arteriosclerosis, Thrombosis, and Vascular Biology, 21*(12), 2072–2079.

Warmerdam, L., van Straten, A., Twisk, J., Riper, H., & Cuijpers, P. (2008). Internet-based treatment for adults with depressive symptoms: Randomized controlled trial. *Journal of Medical Internet Research, 10*, e44.

Wei, W.S. (2013). Time series analysis. https://www.oxfordhandbooks.com/

White, I. R., Carpenter, J., & Horton, N. J. (2012). Including all individuals is not enough: Lessons for intention-to-treat analysis. *Clinical Trials, 9*, 396–407.

Wilson, I. B. (2010). Adherence, placebo effects, and mortality. *Journal of General Internal Medicine, 25*, 1270–1272.

Woertman, W., de Hoop, E., Moerbeek, M., Zuidem, S. U., Gerritsen, D. L., & Teerenstra, S. (2013). Stepped wedge designs could reduce the required sample size in cluster randomized trials. *Journal of Clinical Epidemiology, 66*, 752–758.

Wright, C. C., & Sim, J. (2003). Intention-to-treat approach to data from randomized controlled trials: A sensitivity analysis. *Journal of Clinical Epidemiology, 56*, 833–842.

Zeger, S. L., & Liang, K.-Y. (1986). Longitudinal data analysis for discrete and continuous outcomes. *Biometrics, 42*, 121–130.

Index

Printed in the United States
by Baker & Taylor Publisher Services